DUAL FITNESS: PHYSICAL & SPIRITUAL

A 31-DAY DEVOTIONAL TO BE USED ALONGSIDE YOUR NORMAL FITNESS PROGRAM

Daniel Grell

Photographer: Daniel Grell
Photos: Exercise equipment at stations along fitness trail in Lincoln Park, Chicago, IL

ISBN-13: 978-1518899454
ISBN-10: 1518899455

A special thanks to my wife Gloria who has faithfully wakened with me at 5:00 am each morning so we can meet with God in scripture reading and prayer, and faithfully followed with some kind of regular exercise…thus striving for dual fitness: physical and spiritual.

Table of Contents

Introduction

I began life on November 9, 1949. With that information you can figure out my present age. In my later years most people think I don't look as old as I am. I guess I've been blessed of God with young looking genes. My maternal grandfather lived past his 100th birthday so I guess I've also been blessed with longevity genes. But I believe another reason I don't look my age at this point in my life is I've fairly consistently worked at trying to stay physically fit. Staying fit all these years has not been easy. In fact as I get older, the task seems to get harder. But I discovered a number of years ago one big secret to staying fit was to have a proper understanding of fitness as it relates to who I am in the big picture of life.

Whether you believe you are who you are because of intelligent design or you are who you are based on the theory of evolutionary principles, I think we would all agree that we are unique creatures. There are so many different aspects to who we are; We are multifaceted creatures. We have a physical element to who we are. We touch, see, hear, and move. We are emotional creatures. We laugh, cry, get angry and excited plus many other emotional responses. We are relational, interacting with all kinds of people in many different ways. We have a mental aspect. We think, solve things and we dream. And finally we have a spiritual aspect to us, asking such questions as "Why I'm here?" "What happens when I die?" "How can I be a just person?"

Most who talk about fitness focus mostly on the physical aspect of who we are. Thus, what are talked about are health, exercise routines, diets, and beauty aids. But all these are based on self-gratification and a total focus on self. What's a healthy body going to do for me unless there's some purpose to living? The point is, there's more to life then just me.

There is a book in the Bible called Colossians. In chapter one, verse 16, I read the following words that help me understand the purpose of my being here. The writer says, "…all things were created through him and for him." The "him" being spoken of is Jesus Christ. This reminds me that it is God the Son who created me and I have been created for his use and for his purposes. The writer of Psalm 100:3 solidifies my understanding of this truth, "Know that the Lord, he is God! It is he who made us, and we are his; we are his people, and the sheep of his pasture." You might be wondering why knowing that God created me for his purposes helps me stay fit? It's because I want to be physically fit for anything he would ask me to do and for how ever long it will take.

Staying physically fit takes real commitment, effort, determination, endurance, so knowing there is a purpose for staying fit, greater than just my own enjoyment and how I look, helps me press on with the task. Approaching physical fitness from the viewpoint of intelligent design and knowing one facet of who we are is spiritual is the foundation stone on which this devotional book has been developed.

This devotional book is not meant to be a tool that stands alone in your progress towards physical fitness. It is meant to be added to the other things you are using to either stay fit or achieve fitness and give them greater purpose and therefore greater success. Use this in companion with your exercise routine and your dietary plan.

The Bible version used in this study is the ESV (English Standard Version). Any Bible version can be used but if another version is used please note that because different versions sometimes use different English words, references made to certain words might be different, however the meaning would be the same.

I trust that you will find this devotional book an important and useful tool in getting physically fit and ready to serve the one who created you in whatever he has for you to do and for however long he intends for you to serve him.

Blessings,
Daniel Grell

Meaning of Life

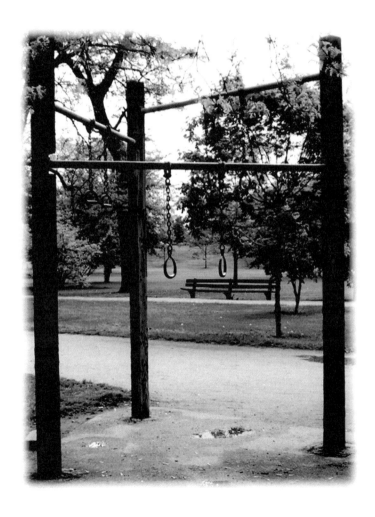

Day 1
Reps and Sets, Without End

<u>Biblical Text:</u> Ecclesiastes 2:1-11

1) I said in my heart, "Come now, I will test you with pleasure; enjoy yourself." But behold, this also was vanity. 2) I said of laughter, "It is mad," and of pleasure, "What use is it?" 3) I searched with my heart how to cheer my body with wine - my heart still guiding me with wisdom - and how to lay hold on folly, till I might see what was good for the children of man to do under heaven during the few days of their life. 4) I made great works. I built houses and planted vineyards for myself. 5) I made myself gardens and parks, and planted in them all kinds of fruit trees. 6) I made myself pools from which to water the forest of growing trees. 7) I bought male and female slaves, and had slaves who were born in my house. I had also great possessions of herds and flocks, more than any who had been before me in Jerusalem. 8) I also gathered for myself silver and gold and the treasure of kings and provinces. I got singers, both men and women, and many concubines, the delight of the children of man.

9) So I became great and surpassed all who were before me in Jerusalem. Also my wisdom remained with me. 10) And whatever my eyes desired I did not keep from them. I kept my heart from no pleasure, for my heart

found pleasure in all my toil, and this was my reward for all my toil. 11) Then I considered all that my hands had done and the toil I had expended in doing it, and behold, all was vanity and a striving after wind, and there was nothing to be gained under the sun.

Theme Verse: Ecclesiastes 2:11 "Then I considered all that my hands had done and the toil I had expended in doing it, and behold, all was vanity and a striving after wind, and there was nothing to be gained under the sun."

Summary: If there was ever a man in history who had it all, who had it made, it was King Solomon, a king who reigned in ancient Israel from 961 to 922 B.C. He was known throughout the world as wise, wealthy, and powerful. His reign was known as the *Golden Age* of Israel. His renown was so great that other rulers travelled great distances to see and experience his greatness. Solomon is known for writing two books in the Bible. The book of Proverbs records his words of wisdom. The other book, Ecclesiastes, seems to be a book that such a man as Solomon would not write. Its theme deals with the vanity of life or as other synonyms define it: futility, emptiness and uselessness. This is Solomon's analysis of his wise, wealthy and powerful life. It was empty.

Observation: Several years ago I saw a bumper sticker that said "Eat Healthy, Exercise Regularly, Die Anyway." These words express in modern day terms what Solomon was feeling. The verses we read today record many of the activities and accomplishments of Solomon. If we were asked to evaluate them we would most likely say, "these were great things he did. Good for him!" But his evaluation of them from verse 11 is that "…all was vanity and a striving after wind, and there was nothing to be gained under the sun." So, what's missing? How is it these activities and accomplishments gain worth? He ends Ecclesiastes with the words in 12:13-14, "The end of the matter; all has been heard. Fear God and keep his commandments, for this is the whole duty of man. For God will bring every deed into judgment, with every secret thing, whether good or evil."

Application: It's easy to feel like Solomon as you repeat endless reps and multiple sets on the dumbbells; as you run mile after mile preparing for a 10K race; as you meticulously weigh, count and record what you had for lunch. Oh, you might feel good about yourself as you buy one size swimsuit smaller than you did last year, cinch your belt one notch tighter than you did last week or looking in the mirror you note with great pride you now have much better muscle definition. But is this all there is after reps, miles and limited lunches? Feel-good moments only last a limited amount of time, if you only keep doing the reps, miles and limited lunches. So where is depth of life to be found? It's in the final words of Solomon, "fear God." This is not being afraid of him, but it is when one acknowledges God for who he is and he is allowed to rule and reign in one's life. It's when one fears God that the reps, miles and limited lunches gain meaning for themselves.

Seeking After God

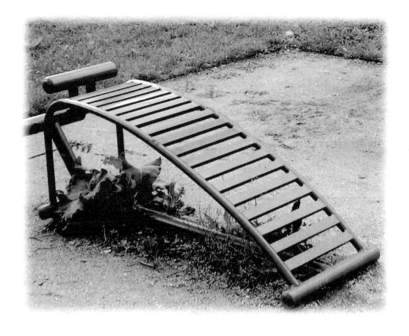

Day 2
Enduring Physical Pain

Biblical Text: Hebrews 12:1-3

> 1) Therefore, since we are surrounded by so great a cloud of witnesses, let us also lay aside every weight, and sin which clings so closely, and let us run with endurance the race that is set before us, 2) looking to Jesus, the founder and perfecter of our faith, who for the joy that was set before him endured the cross, despising the shame, and is seated at the right hand of the throne of God.
> 3) Consider him who endured from sinners such hostility against himself, so that you may not grow weary or fainthearted.

Theme Verse: Hebrews 12:3 "Consider him who endured from sinners such hostility against himself, so that you may not grow weary or fainthearted."

Summary: Hebrews is one of several books in the Bible of unknown authorship. However, though the author is unknown, the focus of the book is certain, the superiority and sufficiency of Jesus in dealing with sin and caring for those who trust in him. This superiority and sufficiency is seen in who he is and what he has done. Hebrews 1:3 says it well "He is the radiance of the glory of God and the exact imprint of his nature, and he upholds the universe by the word of his power. After making purification for sins, he sat down at the right hand of the Majesty on high." Could there be any better words of encouragement given to us?

Observation: It is because of who Jesus is and what he has done with regards to the issue of sin that we can press ahead in life. Though things may trouble us from our past we can move ahead in life without guilt and shame. Not only do we have the declarative description of who Jesus is and what he has done but also 12:1 tells us "Therefore, since we are surrounded by so great a cloud of witnesses…" Who are these witnesses? Chapter 11 gives us a whole list of individuals who had all kinds of challenges in life but pressed ahead because of the promises they had from God. What is required to press ahead? First is to "…lay aside every weight" (vs. 1). Weights can be all kinds of things. It could be the economic and social environment into which we were born and grew up in. It could be a mental, physical, emotional or relational difficulty we've had. But whatever it is we need to "lay aside the weight" and look at Jesus. Why Jesus? Verse 2 spells it out. He did all that was required of him to deal with our troubles. We're also to lay aside "…sin which clings so closely…" (vs. 1). Instead of continuing to sin, which trips us up, or repeating particular sins, which trip us up, we need to "lay aside" the sin and look at Jesus. Why Jesus? Verse 2 spells it out. Notice too that not only has Jesus done all to take care of our troubles and sins but as verse 3 states, he has far surpassed any effort we have given to dealing with our troubles and sins, so look at him, and continue pressing on.

<u>Application:</u> So what does Christ's work of salvation have to do with physical fitness? It comes out in the repeated word "endured." If there was ever a man who faced a physical challenge beyond imagine it was Christ. We're told he endured the cross, so painful a method of execution that the Romans who used it didn't allow citizens of Rome to be crucified. We're also told he endured the hostility of sinners against him. We read in Matthew, Mark, Luke and John how a crown of thorns was pushed down on Jesus' head, he was punched and he was flogged. It's hard to understand how one person could endure such physical pain. And the pain he experienced was the punishment for my sins, which I deserved. So when you're pushing ahead with the final training mile for your marathon, pushing through the added weight on the weight bar to still get the same number of reps as before, striving for one more muscle up in cross-fit, and begin to feel the pain of the added effort, remember the one who suffered so greatly for you. It truly is something to marvel at. We choose to suffer for our own good and glory while Christ suffered, not for himself, but for you and me. He paid the price; he endured the pain of the cross that you and I might be freed from the pain and punishment of our sin.

Day 3
Cheating Death

Biblical Text: 1 Corinthians 15:20-24, 42-49

20) But in fact Christ has been raised from the dead, the first fruits of those who have fallen asleep. 21) For as by a man came death, by a man has come also the resurrection of the dead. 22) For as in Adam all die, so also in Christ shall all be made alive. 23) But each in his own order: Christ the first fruits, then at his coming those who belong to Christ. 24) Then comes the end, when he delivers the kingdom to God the Father after destroying every rule and every authority and power.

42) So is it with the resurrection of the dead. What is sown is perishable; what is raised is imperishable. 43) It is sown in dishonor, it is raised in glory. It is sown in weakness; it is raised in power. 44) It is sown a natural body; it is raised a spiritual body. If there is a natural body, there is also a spiritual body. 45) Thus it is written, "The first man Adam became a living being"; the last Adam became a life-giving spirit.

Theme Verse: 1 Corinthians 15:42 "So is it with the resurrection of the dead. What is sown is perishable; what is raised is imperishable."

Summary: 1 Corinthians is one of two letters written by the Apostle Paul to the followers of Jesus Christ who lived in Corinth, a town in Greece. One of the reasons for Paul writing these two letters was to deal with ethical, moral and theological errors. One of the theological errors he had to confront was an incorrect understanding of the resurrection of Jesus Christ from the dead, following his death on the cross and his burial in the tomb. Chapter 15 of this letter directly attacks this theological error. The necessity of correcting this error is that an incorrect understanding of the resurrection is a direct attack on the Gospel. What is the Gospel? It's very "good news." Paul gives a very clear presentation of the Gospel in the first eleven verses of chapter 15. First, Christ died for our sins. Second, Christ was buried. Third, Christ was resurrected. These three events are the "Good News:" Christ died, he paid the blood price required; Christ was buried, he took the punishment by going to hell; Christ rose, he conquered death. The theological error in Corinth was that some people were saying there is no resurrection. But if that is the case then as Paul puts it in verses 17-19, "And if Christ has not been raised, your faith is futile and you are still in your sins. Then those also who have fallen asleep in Christ have perished. If in this life only we have hope in Christ, we are of all people most to be pitied."

Observation: Our text for today does not argue for the resurrection but takes it as truth and addresses the results of the resurrection. The first truth is that Christ's resurrection is only the beginning of resurrections. His resurrection makes it possible for those who are followers of Jesus Christ to also be resurrected from the dead (vs. 20-23). Secondly, this resurrection ushers out the old world order of world rulers and begins anew under the reign of Christ (vs. 24-28). Thirdly, the resurrection of Jesus Christ abolishes death (vs. 26). Fourth, the resurrection changes our bodies from being perishable to imperishable, from being bodies of weakness to bodies of power (vs. 43), from being earthy bodies to heavenly bodies (vs. 49). This is much of what fitness is all about, trying to change the body into something else, bodies that aren't sickly but healthy, bodies that aren't weak but strong, and bodies that look "heavenly," perfect, toned, muscled, lasting...and bodies that withstand the coming of death for as long as possible.

Application: There are a lot of things in the world of fitness that claim the offer of a heavenly body, one that is perfect, toned, muscled and lasting. Classes, supplements, certain exercises and equipment all make this claim. And while the things they offer can give us what we might think is a more heavenly body, the truth is it's only a temporary fix. None of the things they offer have defeated death. Death for all of us is only a matter of time and that's why we need to get prepared for it. Yes, keep death at bay by staying fit, but ultimately defeat the results of death by believing the "Good News," Christ died for your sins, Christ was buried and Christ rose from the dead defeating death. So you want that heavenly body? Jesus Christ is the only one who can give it to you. Give your life to him. Allow him to rule and reign in your earthly body.

Day 4
Fearless in the Battle

Biblical Text: 2 Samuel 23:8-12

8) These are the names of the mighty men whom David had: Josheb-basshebeth a Tahche-monite; he was chief of the three. He wielded his spear against eight hundred whom he killed at one time.

9) And next to him among the three mighty men was Eleazar the son of Dodo, son of Ahohi. He was with David when they defied the Philistines who were gathered there for battle, and the men of Israel withdrew. 10) He rose and struck down the Philistines until his hand was weary, and his hand clung to the sword. And the Lord brought about a great victory that day, and the men returned after him only to strip the slain.

11) And next to him was Shammah, the son of Agee the Hararite. The Philistines gathered together at Lehi, where there was a plot of ground full of lentils, and the men fled from the Philistines. 12) But he took his stand in the midst of the plot and defended it and struck down the Philistines, and the Lord worked a great victory.

Theme Verse: 2 Samuel 23:12b "...and the Lord worked a great victory."

Summary: The book of 1 Samuel covers the historical account of Israel moving from a theocracy (governed by God) to being governed by their first King, Saul. 1 Samuel also details how King Saul turns from obedience to God and loses his kingdom to the young man named David, who is also introduced to us in 1 Samuel. A quick reading of 1 Samuel shows David's ascension to the throne of Israel, though promised to him by God, is not an easy road. His ascension finally takes place with King Saul's death at the end of 1 Samuel. 2 Samuel is the historical record of King David's reign and rule, the good and the bad, the blessings and the challenges.

Observation: Throughout the reading of 1 and 2 Samuel the story about David includes many other individuals. It was these individuals who God used to help David through the struggles of life and ascension to the thrown. Our text introduces three men, their heritage, and their difficult names to pronounce, Josheb-basshebeth a Tahchemonite, Eleazar the son of Dodo, son of Ahohite, and finally, Shammah the son Agee the Hararite. While their heritage and names might be interesting it is the description of what they were like and what they did we want to focus on. Verse 8 describes them as "…the mighty men whom David had…" The Hebrew word "might" has various meanings. It can mean strong, brave, and or mighty. Looking at what they did makes us think there was an element of all three meanings. Josheb-basshebeth, slew 800 hundred men in one battle. Eleazar, stood the course of battle to victory when everyone else retreated. It was no doubt a hard and fierce fight as it says his hand became so weary at the end he couldn't even open it to let go of the sword. Shammah, also stood his ground in a field of lentils to defeat the enemy even when everyone else fled. When standing alone in a battle it helps to be physically fit. Strength and size help win the battle because they're good for intimidation.

Application: While it looks like these men were alone in their battle and only because of their strength, bravery and might won the battles that confronted them, they actually had a helper. Verse 10 says, "and the Lord brought about a great victory…" and verse 12 says, "…and the Lord worked a great victory." This is a very important truth to understand. The Lord, our creator God, is not only the one who enables us to have victory in our battles but he also gives us great victories. So for the battles of life, how do I get the strength, bravery and might of these three men? Strength and might come from getting physically fit and pumping iron. Then you can endure the length of the battle and the blows in the battle. But is strength and might sufficient for the battles of life? Probably not. What we need added to strength and might is bravery. But where does bravery come from? I think our text clarifies it for us in the statements "and the Lord brought about a great victory" (vs. 10) and "the Lord worked a great victory" (vs. 12). When facing a battle I want to know someone is with me. In fact I want someone greater than my strength and might which have a limit. I want the omnipotent strength and power of God for he alone is the one who gives victory. Work hard to get strength and might. But seek the Lord God to gain bravery. Invite him to join you in the battles of life you face and experience victory.

Day 5
Be Willing to Climb a Tree

<u>Biblical Text:</u> Luke 19:1-10

1) He entered Jericho and was passing through. 2) And there was a man named Zacchaeus. He was a chief tax collector and was rich. 3) And he was seeking to see who Jesus was, but on account of the crowd he could not, because he was small of stature. 4) So he ran on ahead and climbed up into a sycamore tree to see him, for he was about to pass that way. 5) And when Jesus came to the place, he looked up and said to him, "Zacchaeus, hurry and come down, for I must stay at your house today." 6) So he hurried and came down and received him joyfully. 7) And when they saw it, they all grumbled, "He has gone in to be the guest of a man who is a sinner." 8) And Zacchaeus stood and said to the Lord, "Behold, Lord, the half of my goods I give to the poor. And if I have defrauded anyone of anything, I restore it fourfold." 9) And Jesus said to him, "Today salvation has come to this house, since he also is a son of Abraham. For the Son of Man came to seek and to save the lost."

<u>Theme Verse:</u> Luke 19:3 "And he was seeking to see who Jesus was, but on account of the crowd he could not, because he was small of stature."

Summary: Today we are introduced to a man named Zaccheus. Today he would be called Zach. Zach had done well in life. He had advanced to upper management in the tax office of Jericho. Verse 8 would lead us to believe that he had become very wealthy, since he had sufficient money to fund a major project assisting the poor. Though he had position and wealth, he had some challenges: people didn't like him (vs. 7) and he was short (vs. 2). When Jesus came to town, nothing kept Zach from doing all he needed to do to see Jesus, which led to his connecting with Jesus, which led to a life transformed by Jesus.

Observation: Jesus was an important man to meet. Zach probably didn't know how important a man Jesus was, or the effect that he could have on his life. We don't know what he knew about Jesus, but he was not about to let things stand in the way of his getting to see him. Many things could have stood in his way. Pride that could come from position and wealth: "Me climb a tree? I'm above that." An unwillingness to deal with a physical issue that stood in his way: "Me climb a tree? I'm physically unable to do that," or "I don't want to admit that I'm short." No! Jesus needed to be encountered, and nothing was going to stand in Zach's way.

Application: For some of you, Jesus is someone you need to meet. For others of you, Jesus is someone you already know, but you never got to know him really well. There can be many reasons why, but the bottom line is that we allow things to stand in our way. Sometimes they are prideful reasons (I'm too important). Sometimes they are negative reasons (I don't like myself and the way Jesus made me). Jesus is too important not to meet him and get to know him really well. He is coming to town soon, so be a Zach and do whatever you need to do to overcome the things that stand in the way of having a transformed life with Jesus. What do you need to overcome?

Day 6
A Selling Point

Biblical Text: Romans 12:1-2

> 1) I appeal to you therefore, brothers, by the mercies of God, to present your bodies as a living sacrifice, holy and acceptable to God, which is your spiritual worship. 2) Do not be conformed to this world, but be transformed by the renewal of your mind, that by testing you may discern what is the will of God, what is good and acceptable and perfect.

Theme Verse: Romans 12:1 "I appeal to you therefore, brothers, by the mercies of God, to present your bodies as a living sacrifice, holy and acceptable to God, which is your spiritual worship."

Summary: A man named Paul wrote the New Testament book of Romans. It was a letter written to Christians who lived in the city of Rome. As is typical of Paul's letters, it has two parts. The first part deals with doctrine or what might be called Christian truth. It goes from chapter one through the end of chapter eleven. The second part is from Romans 12:1 to the end of the book. It deals with practical Christian living. It's important to know that the second part is based on the first part. The is the reason that Paul begins with the words "I appeal to you therefore, brothers, by the mercies of God…" What Paul is now going to talk about is grounded in the mercies of God described in the first part which tells us Jesus Christ took the punishment for our sins so that God will no longer condemn us for our sins. This is a gift to us from God if we receive this gift. Now in response we give ourselves completely to God.

Observation: It's not unusual when challenging someone to do something, buy something, or commit to something you present to them a reason for the challenge. This also holds true for fitness. Do you remember why you bought that ab machine advertized on T.V that now sits in your garage collecting dust? It was because the demonstrator of the machine was lean and fit and displayed abs you wished you had. No one said they used the machine to get that way. You were allowed to assume that through their demonstration. And so you sacrificed your budget and agreed to pay the three payments of $19.99. Most things related to fitness, be it equipment, clothing, books or magazines, always focus, generally by picture, on a fit person, through using the advertized items, the body you can have.

Application: There are many things calling for us to give a sacrifice to them. Gym memberships, appropriate equipment and clothing, all call us to sacrifice our finances. Exercise and training ask us to sacrifice our time. Diets and supplements ask us to sacrifice our palate. But what have these things done for us? Nothing that lasts! So when thinking of sacrifices you need to make to achieve fitness, make sure you first sacrifice (give yourself fully) to one who has done something for you that is lasting, Jesus

Christ, who has given his all that you might be fit for God.

Day 7
Confronting Hurdles

Biblical Text: Psalm 18:25-29

25) With the merciful you show yourself
merciful;
with the blameless man you show
yourself blameless;
26) with the purified you show yourself
pure;
and with the crooked you make
yourself tortuous.
27) For you save a humble people,
but the haughty eyes you bring down.
28) For it is you who light my lamp;
the Lord my God lightens my
darkness.
29) For by you I can run against a troop,
and by my God I can leap over a wall.

Theme Verse: Psalm 18:29
"For by you I can run against a troop,
and by my God I can leap over a wall."

Summary: The book of Psalms is one of the books in the Bible where the words written are the heart cry of the writer. They are the emotional outpouring of the writer. Sometimes they are words of joy or happiness, sometimes they are words that indicate the writer was depressed or discouraged. While the words of the Psalm might tell us the emotional condition of the writer, it's not always easy to know why they were feeling a particular way. However some of the Psalms do tell us. Psalm 18 is one of the Psalms that tells us why the writer was so positive. David, expressing his great joy, wrote how the Lord had delivered him from all his enemies, including King Saul who had been hunting him down for a long time.

Observation: This verse clearly indicates David has a great trust in God. His trust is in a God who is so mighty and powerful that he can help him have victory over any difficulty. This verse tells us that David can even trust God to help him crush a whole army. And the wall that he can jump over would indicate any kind of major difficulty. There is no one individual, no group or situation that with God's help he will not have victory. This is a wonderful truth to know, God can help us have victory over any trouble that might come our way. Victory does not come from our abilities but from God.

Application: What helps you be a conqueror and enable you to achieve any hurdle before you? In the physical realm there are many things we use to assure victories. In physical events like cross fit competition we would engage in strength training, and cardio development. Safety on the streets would direct us to judo, taekwondo and other self-defense type classes. A desire for high level sports positions might find us attending summer sports camps and hiring personal coaches. While all those might be good things for us they only address the physical challenges. But remember you are also a mental, emotional, relational and spiritual being. Who or what will give you victories in the wars and challenges of these areas? King David can answer that for you. It is God. Look to the one who alone can help you win the battles of life and press through the hurdles of life.

Day 8
The Secret of Endurance

<u>Biblical Text:</u> Isaiah 40:27-31

27) Why do you say, O Jacob,
        and speak, O Israel,
      "My way is hidden from the Lord,
        and my right is disregarded by my
          God"?
28) Have you not known? Have you not
          heard?
      The Lord is the everlasting God,
        the Creator of the ends of the earth.
      He does not faint or grow weary;
        his understanding is unsearchable.
29) He gives power to the faint,
        and to him who has no might he
          increases strength.
30) Even youths shall faint and be weary,
        and young men shall fall exhausted;
31) but they who wait for the Lord shall
          renew their strength;
        they shall mount up with wings like
          eagles;
      they shall run and not be weary;
        they shall walk and not faint.

<u>Theme Verse:</u> Isaiah 40:31
      "but they who wait for the Lord shall
          renew their strength;
      they shall mount up with wings like
          eagles;

> they shall run and not be weary;
> they shall walk and not faint."

Summary: The book of Isaiah is the written record of the vision of a prophet named Isaiah. Isaiah lived and prophesied during the reigns of numerous kings of Judah: Uzziah, Jotham, Ahaz and Hezekiah. God used Isaiah to proclaim the greatness of God and to speak against the sins of his people. In our text for today Isaiah is speaking against a false notion these people had. They thought God would not know about their sins and would therefore not punish them. Isaiah refutes this thinking by declaring God's unfailing greatness. It is also this unfailing greatness that helps his faithful followers endure.

Observation: Our text for today makes a true statement in verse 30, "Even youths shall faint and be weary, and young men shall fall exhausted. "Doesn't matter how young or vigorous, at some point everyone wears out. As I've worked at an increased level of fitness I've discovered it's a lot about endurance. Longer races require greater endurance. Heavier weights require greater endurance. Limiting food requires greater endurance. All aspects of fitness require one to have greater endurance as the challenge increases. The thing is, at some point endurance eventually gives out. Even the super athlete who does the endurance sport of 100 mile runs and full Ironman triathlons eventually gives out. That's why Isaiah points to God. He alone who is omnipotent (all powerful), everlasting and creator of all things does not become tired or weary.

Application: Life is made up of several different parts. There are the physical, emotional, mental, relational and spiritual parts of who we are. Each must be dealt with differently. Go ahead and do all you can with regards the physical man. Make sure you do what it takes to stay fit. But when it comes to the emotional, relational and spiritual areas you can't make it on your own. Unless God is allowed to be involved in your life in a significant way you will become weary and tired. So, wait on God, he alone can give you new strength, keep you from getting tired and growing weary.

Day 9
Winning

Biblical Text: Genesis 32:22-32

22) The same night he arose and took his two wives, his two female servants, and his eleven children, and crossed the ford of the Jabbok. 23) He took them and sent them across the stream, and everything else that he had. 24) And Jacob was left alone. And a man wrestled with him until the breaking of the day. 25) When the man saw that he did not prevail against Jacob, he touched his hip socket, and Jacob's hip was put out of joint as he wrestled with him. 26) Then he said, "Let me go, for the day has broken." But Jacob said, "I will not let you go unless you bless me." 27) And he said to him, "What is your name?" And he said, "Jacob." 28) Then he said, "Your name shall no longer be called Jacob, but Israel, for you have striven with God and with men, and have prevailed. 29) Then Jacob asked him, "Please tell me your name." But he said "Why is it that you ask my name?" And there he blessed him. 30) So Jacob called the name of the place Peniel, saying, "For I have seen God face to face, and yet my life has been delivered." 31) The sun rose upon him as he passed Penuel, limping because of his hip. 32) Therefore to this day the people of Israel do not eat the sinew of the thigh that is on the hip socket,

because he touched the socket of Jacob's hip on the sinew of the thigh.

Theme Verse: Genesis 32:26 "Then he said, 'Let me go, for the day has broken.' But Jacob said, 'I will not let you go unless you bless me.' "

Summary: We enter this story in the middle of Jacob's return trip to his home. Years earlier Jacob had cheated his brother Esau out of his inheritance and blessing, so he had to flee to his uncle Laban's home to save his life. During Jacob's stay at his uncle's home, he too experienced being cheated out of what was due him, but he gained wealth and two wives. Hoping that years have healed his brother's feelings toward him, he makes the return journey to his home. One night on the journey he meets God and has a wrestling match with him. His goal? Win the match and get a blessing.

Observation: It seems as though Jacob's life is an example of fighting hard for what you want. His fighting was not always a model of fairness, but it is a model of striving hard to get what you want. He fought hard and did what he needed to, in order to get the family inheritance, the father's blessing, his uncle's wealth, and his wives. This is a model of winning, but not a model about how to win.

Application: Much of fitness is about fighting. We fight the "battle of the bulge." We fight and strain to do one more pull-up. We fight against pain when training for a triathlon. It takes a real fighter to win these battles. But there are more battles to fight than just the fitness battle. Be a Jacob. Grab hold of God and wrestle with him, hanging onto him until you find blessing from him.

Lordship

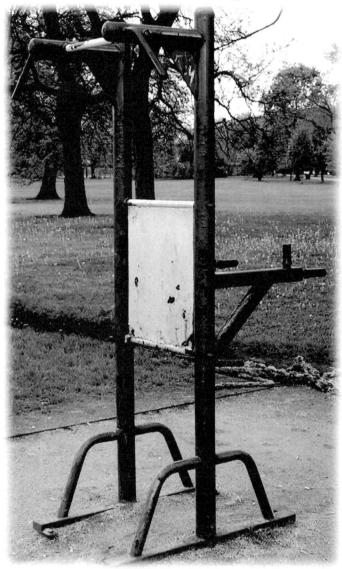

Day 10
Valued

Biblical Text: Psalm 147:1-20

1) Praise the Lord!
For it is good to sing praises to
our God;
for it is pleasant, and a song of praise
is fitting.
2) The Lord builds up Jerusalem;
he gathers the outcasts of Israel.
3) He heals the brokenhearted
and binds up their wounds.
4) He determines the number of the stars;
he gives to all of them their names.
5) Great is our Lord, and abundant in
power;
his understanding is beyond measure.
6) The Lord lifts up the humble;
he casts the wicked to the ground.

7) Sing to the Lord with thanksgiving;
make melody to our God on the lyre!
8) He covers the heavens with clouds;
he prepares rain for the earth;
he makes grass grow on the hills.
9) He gives to the beasts their food,
and to the young ravens that cry.
10) His delight is not in the strength of the
horse,
nor his pleasure in the legs of a man,
11) but the Lord takes pleasure in those

who fear him,
in those who hope in his steadfast
love.

12) Praise the Lord, O Jerusalem!
Praise your God, O Zion!
13) For he strengthens the bars of your
gates;
he blesses your children within you.
14) He makes peace in your borders;
he fills you with the finest of the
wheat.
15) He sends out his command to the
earth;
his word runs swiftly.
16) He gives snow like wool;
he scatters hoarfrost like ashes.
17) He hurls down his crystals of ice like
crumbs;
who can stand before his cold?
18) He sends out his word, and melts
them;
he makes his wind blow and the
waters flow.
19) He declares his word to Jacob,
his statutes and rules to Israel.
20) He has not dealt thus with any other
nation;
they do not know his rules.
Praise the Lord."

Theme Verse: Psalm 147:11
"but the Lord takes pleasure in those

who fear him,
in those who hope in his steadfast
love."

Summary: This psalm is written after a period of time when the people of Jerusalem had experienced great defeat, suffering and sorrow. We don't know exactly what had happened to bring these things about but these times were now at an end. The writer expresses the ends to these times with words like "the Lord builds up" (vs. 2), and "He heals the brokenhearted and binds up their wounds" (vs. 3). How is it possible that God can bring about this restoration and healing? The writer directs us to God's great power and might as seen in his active work of caring for his created world. Notice in verses 8 - 9 how he brings rain upon the earth, which in turn causes the grass to grow which then provides food for all the animals. Notice how he is described as the cause of weather in verses 15 - 18. He is the one who controls the snow, the frost, the hailstones, the cold, and the wind. All these things display God's power and thus ability to intervene in desperate situations.

Observation It's interesting to note that though God is truly omnipotent (all powerful) as seen in his control of the weather and restoring a defeated people, it isn't power and strength with which he is impressed. Verse 10 expresses his thoughts, "His delight is not in the strength of the horse, nor his pleasure in the legs of a man." God definitely thinks differently than I do and most around me. Having not spent much time around horses other than a few hour long trail rides over the years, I can't comment on the strength they have other than express my amazement as to how easily they carry my 200 pound frame over the roughest of terrains. But go to the gym and I do find myself impressed with how some young men have developed their bodies. I also note they too are somewhat impressed with their strength as they flex and pose in front of the mirrors that adorn the wall. So if this all powerful God is not impressed with the strength of men, since it pales in all ways to his power, what does God take note of? Verse 11 tells us what God values are those who fear him and put their hope in him.

Application: Next time you're at the gym and note the massive biceps and powerful pecs being flexed around you, guard yourself from being overly impressed. Yes, it would be nice to have a well developed physique, but let me tell you, no matter how hard you try and how well developed you become, it all eventually begins to sag, to become less defined. In the eyes of the world you may begin to feel less value in who you are, but take note of this. There is one who takes great value in you. It is the one who is all-powerful as displayed by controlling the weather and restoring those who are broken. Feeling a little undervalued in the gym or on the sports team because your biceps don't compare to others around you, your physical ability doesn't compare to others? Find your value in the eyes of your Creator. How does that happen? First as verse 11 says, "fear him," which means to put him first place in your life and second "…hope in his steadfast love."

Day 11
Worshipping a False God

Biblical Text: Exodus 20:1-17

1) And God spoke all these words, saying,

2) "I am the Lord your God, who brought you out of the land of Egypt, out of the house of slavery.

3) "You shall have no other gods before me.

4) "You shall not make for yourself a carved image, or any likeness of anything that is in heaven above, or that is in the earth beneath, or that is in the water under the earth. 5) You shall not bow down to them or serve them, for I the Lord your God am a jealous God, visiting the iniquity of the fathers on the children to the third and the fourth generation of those who hate me, 6) but showing steadfast love to thousands of those who love me and keep my commandments.

7) "You shall not take the name of the Lord your God in vain, for the Lord will not hold him guiltless who takes his name in vain.

8) "Remember the Sabbath day, to keep it holy. 9) Six days you shall labor, and do all your work, 10) but the seventh day is a Sabbath to the Lord your God. On it you shall not do any work, you, or your son, or your daughter, your male servant, or your female servant, or your livestock, or the sojourner who is within

your gates. 11) For in six days the Lord made heaven and earth, the sea, and all that is in them, and rested the seventh day. Therefore the Lord blessed the Sabbath day and made it holy.

12) "Honor your father and your mother, that your days may be long in the land that the Lord your God is giving you.

13) "You shall not murder.

14) "You shall not commit adultery.

15) "You shall not steal.

16) "You shall not bear false witness against your neighbor.

17) "You shall not covet your neighbor's house; you shall not covet your neighbor's wife, or his male servant, or his female servant, or his ox, or his donkey, or anything that is your neighbor's."

Theme Verse: Exodus 20:3 "You shall have no other gods before me."

Summary: The book of Exodus is the historical account of how God rescues a group of people out of slavery in Egypt, builds them into a nation and starts the process of taking them to a new land he has promised to give them. The people are those who claim Abraham, Isaac and Jacob as their forefathers. They moved from the land of Canaan because of a famine during the days of Jacob. When they moved to Egypt they entered the land as a small family group but now exiting Egypt they leave as a large multitude of diverse families. Before they get back to Canaan,

God needs some nation building time since they've been ruled the last 430 years by Egyptian authorities. Now, on their own, they need new leaders, structures and laws to guide them. In order to do this God has brought them to a place on their journey called Mount Sinai. It is here he begins to build them into a nation. The governing structure he has for them is called a "theocracy." This means they will be a nation and people that are ruled by God and not by man.

Observation: Our text of today records the Ten Commandments God gives to his people to establish his theocracy and to guide his people. The first four give direction regarding their relationship with God; the last six give direction regarding their relationship with other people. If God is the supreme ruler of this people then it's not hard to understand why the first two commandments put him at the top of things, with nothing else allowed to become first place, a higher priority, or more time and effort given to them. That which is important to us as well as gives direction to our life needs to be given top priority. Physical fitness requires this too. If you are going to be physically fit and do all that is required to be fit you have to give it a significant place in your life. If not, it just isn't going to happen. The busyness of life created by work, family, and obligations are going to sap the necessary time fitness takes. Fitness needs high priority on the "to do" list and the budget if it's going to happen.

Application: But wait a minute! While personal physical fitness is good, important and even fun, do we really want to elevate it to the level of a "god?" A god who controls our time, finances, relationships, our very being? If not to the level of a god, to at least the level of making personal physical fitness an "idol?" An idol to which we give allegiance and allow to be a major influencer of what we do and how we live? So if fitness is a very important aspect of my life, important for health and service to God, and the only way it will be accomplished is to make it a major discipline in my life, giving time and finances to it, how do I keep it from being an idol or elevating it to the level of a god in my life? The first thing is to keep it in proper perspective by following God's first two commands, "You shall have no other gods before me" (vs. 3), and "You shall not make for yourself a carved image, or any likeness of anything that is in heaven above, or that is in the earth beneath, or that is in the water under the earth" (vs. 4). Having our creator God in his proper place and following his rule will always keep us balanced in our life. Also, keeping personal fitness as a priority doesn't mean control. It just means that it's kept as an important element of our life, included in the process of decision-making but will allow for flexibility when needed and not just the controlling element of our life.

Day 12
The Danger of Buff

Biblical Text: Genesis 39:1-23

1) Now Joseph had been brought down to Egypt, and Potiphar, an officer of Pharaoh, the captain of the guard, an Egyptian, had bought him from the Ishmaelites who had brought him down there. 2) The Lord was with Joseph, and he became a successful man, and he was in the house of his Egyptian master. 3) His master saw that the Lord was with him and that the Lord caused all that he did to succeed in his hands. 4) So Joseph found favor in his sight and attended him, and he made him overseer of his house and put him in charge of all that he had. 5) From the time that he made him overseer in his house and over all that he had the Lord blessed the Egyptian's house for Joseph's sake; the blessing of the Lord was on all that he had, in house and field. 6) So he left all that he had in Joseph's charge, and because of him he had no concern about anything but the food he ate.

Now Joseph was handsome in form and appearance. 7) And after a time his master's wife cast her eyes on Joseph and said, "Lie with me." 8) But he refused and said to his master's wife, "Behold, because of me my master has no concern about anything in the house, and he has put everything that he has in my charge. 9) He is not greater in this house than I am, nor has he kept back anything from me except yourself, because you are his wife. How then can I do this great wickedness and sin against God?" 10) And as she spoke to Joseph day after day, he would not listen to her, to lie beside her or to be with her.

11) But one day, when he went into the house to do his work and none of the men of the house was there in the house, 12) she caught him by his garment, saying, "Lie with me." But he left his garment in her hand and fled and got out of the house. 13) And as soon as she saw that he had left his garment in her hand and had fled out of the house, 14) she called to the men of her household and said to them, "See, he has brought among us a Hebrew to laugh at us. He came in to me to lie with me, and I cried out with a loud voice. 15) And as soon as he heard that I lifted up my voice and cried out, he left his garment beside me and fled and got out of the house." 16) Then she laid up his garment by her until his master came home, 17) and she told him the same story, saying, "The Hebrew servant, whom you have brought among us, came in to me to laugh at me. 18) But as soon as I lifted up my voice and cried, he left his garment beside me and fled out of the house."

19) As soon as his master heard the words that his wife spoke to him, "This is the way your servant treated me," his anger was kindled. 20) And Joseph's master took him and put him into the prison, the place where the

king's prisoners were confined, and he was there in prison. 21) But the lord was with Joseph and showed him steadfast love and gave him favor in the sight of the keeper of the prison. 22) And the keeper of the prison put Joseph in charge of all the prisoners who were in the prison. Whatever was done there, he was the one who did it. 23) The keeper of the prison paid no attention to anything that was in Joseph's charge, because the Lord was with him. And whatever he did the Lord made it succeed.

Theme Verse: Genesis 39:6 "...Now Joseph was handsome in form and appearance."

Summary: If there is one thing the life of Joseph teaches us it is that no matter how hard things may be, if you focus on obedience to God, he will help you pull through. Our text begins with the results of Joseph's brothers' jealousy toward him. If you don't know about their jealousy, read Genesis 38. Because of their jealousy, they have sold him to slave traders. Slavery is a horrible situation to find yourself in. The slave traders sell him in the slave markets of Egypt to a man named Potiphar. Because of Joseph's faithfulness to God, God blesses him as he serves in Potiphar's house. His service is so commendable that Potiphar puts him in charge of everything. The description of Joseph is that he is good-looking and buff. This stud of a young man attracts the attention of Potiphar's wife who desiring him wants him to sleep with her. He refuses. She in spite, lies, which results in Potiphar getting rid of him. Now instead of a slave he is in the deep dungeons of Pharaoh's prison system. But again God blesses his faithfulness by impressing the chief jailer who puts him in a position of managing the jail.

Observation: Of the many reasons we care about how we look so that we exercise and diet, one is certainly that we care about how other people perceive us. There is no place in the text that indicates Joseph spent any time doing these things or even thought about them. As a slave you didn't have time to think about yourself. Slavery was a life of hard physical work. But it was probably the hard physical work as a slave added on to an already fit life having been a shepherd boy for his father that made him the stud of the man he was. It's not unusual if good-looking and having a good physique that people notice you. But notice the response to Potiphar's wife as she throws herself at him, "…How then can I do this great wickedness and sin against God?" (vs. 9). This young man has a correct perspective of who he is. He knows without a doubt that the reason he looks the way he does is for the purposes of God. Thus, instead of succumbing to the sexual advance of this woman as many might, he keeps his focus on God.

Application: So, you finally like how you look. You've faithfully pumped iron, done your aerobics and watched your diet. Hitting the beach you triumphantly take off your shirt and wait to see everyone fall down in worshipful awe of the stud you've become. But something happens that you didn't expect, overtures of sexual interest are made towards you. It's at this very moment you need to decide what life is all about. Is it the body you've made yourself to be or is it something deeper than this, like being one who has been created in the image of God and desires to please God in all things. Though the buff body is nice to have, "It ain't gonna last." The only thing that will last is your relationship with God. It is he who brings true blessing, not the buff body.

Spiritual Growth

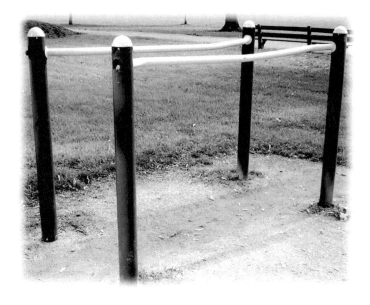

Day 13
Preparing for the Climb

Biblical Text: Psalm 121:1-8

1) I lift up my eyes to the hills.
    From where does my help come?
2) My help comes from the Lord,
    who made heaven and earth.

3) He will not let your foot be moved;
    he who keeps you will not slumber.
4) Behold, he who keeps Israel
    will neither slumber nor sleep.

5) The Lord is your keeper;
    the Lord is your shade on your right
        hand.
6) The sun shall not strike you by day,
    nor the moon by night.

7) The Lord will keep you from all evil;
    he will keep your life.
8) The Lord will keep
    your going out and your coming in
    from this time forth and forevermore.

Theme Verse: Psalm 121:1-2
    "I lift up my eyes to the hills.
        From where does my help come?
    My help comes from the Lord,
        who made heaven and earth.

Summary: The Book of Psalms can be called the Hymn Book and Prayer Book of the Israelites. Psalm 120 through 134 is a group of psalms known as the "Songs of Ascents." It is thought these psalms were sung by those taking a spiritual journey to Jerusalem. Since Jerusalem is located on top of a hill, most people making the journey have to ascend, or walk uphill. This psalm tells of a traveler who is far off. As he looks ahead to the mountain journey, which he has to make, he begins to think of all the possible dangers ahead, dangerous terrain, possible robbers, and the heat of the day. Thinking of these things causes him to be well prepared for all the possibilities of trouble, but in the end, no matter how well one is prepared, things still happen. This traveler knows that ultimately he must put his life into the loving hands of his sovereign Creator, the mountain maker.

Observation: Over the years I've learned from one of my sons, who loves rock-climbing, the importance of adequate preparation and appropriate safety equipment. As he climbs up the side of the mountain, he needs such things as helmet, ropes, and pitons. He needs sufficient water, nutrition, and strength. He also needs to have had sufficient instruction in the sport, and finally to gain experience before he progresses to more difficult climbs.

Application: It can be said that any sport needs adequate preparation and appropriate safety equipment. But this can also be said about anything in life, including the spiritual life. How does one adequately prepare for the spiritual journey? Try Bible reading. Where does one find appropriate safety for the journey? Try finding a Bible-teaching church, a Bible study, and someone to disciple or mentor you. But begin the journey by lifting up your eyes to the One who made the mountains, God the creator.

Day 14
A Trophy Winner

Biblical Text: 1 Corinthians 9:24-27

> 24) Do you not know that in a race all the runners compete, but only one receives the prize? So run that you may obtain it. 25) Every athlete exercises self-control in all things. They do it to receive a perishable wreath, but we an imperishable. 26) So I do not run aimlessly; I do not box as one beating the air. 27) But I discipline my body and keep it under control, lest after preaching to others I myself should be disqualified.

Theme Verse: I Corinthians 9:25 "Every athlete exercises self-control in all things. They do it to receive a perishable wreath, but we an imperishable."

Summary: It was not unusual for the authors of Scripture to use examples and illustrations from sports. Sports were something with which the ancient Greeks and Romans were familiar. The Olympic games began in Greece, and the Romans built stadiums wherever they conquered, so that they could have chariot races and gladiatorial games. In our text, today, Paul is teaching the Christians who lived in the city of Corinth what they needed to do in order to introduce Jesus Christ to those who did not know him as their Savior. Since people were all different, different approaches needed to be taken. It's just like sports. In order to win the event, you need to do the right kind of training for it. And it takes just as much training and discipline to live a life that presents Christ to others as it does to run a race to win or box to have a KO.

Observation: Having most of my life generally worked at fitness, at the ripe old age of fifty-eight, I decided that it was time to compete in a triathlon. I soon discovered that my general commitment to recreational swimming, bike riding, running, and strength training was not sufficient if I was going to finish the triathlon sprint distance (1/2 mile swim, 17-mile bike, 3-mile run). I had to discipline my body and keep it under control. It took much more than just wishing to compete in the triathlon, for that just doesn't get the body out of bed in the morning to jump into cold water. Whatever sport you do, wanting it to move from recreational to competitive requires some very specific things to take place. You need self-control (vs. 25), run with aim (the setting of goals) (vs. 26) and discipline (vs. 27). These three things are essential if you want to win in your sport.

Application: Paul uses the illustration of sport to teach us what needs to happen if we want to win an earthly prize (vs. 25). Just think how much self-control, setting of goals, and discipline top athletes give to win prizes that soon fade. If this is done for fading prizes, shouldn't we who want lasting prizes, God's riches in heaven, engage in these same things in our spiritual life? Are you content with being just a recreational Christian, or do you want to be a winning Christian? Apply self-control, the setting of goals, and discipline to your walk with Christ.

Day 15
Taking Control of Your Body

<u>Biblical Text:</u> 1 Corinthians 9:24-27

> 24) Do you not know that in a race all the runners compete, but only one receives the prize? So run that you may obtain it. 25) Every athlete exercises self-control in all things. They do it to receive a perishable wreath, but we an imperishable. 26) So I do not run aimlessly; I do not box as one beating the air. 27) But I discipline my body and keep it under control, lest after preaching to others I myself should be disqualified.

<u>Theme Verse:</u> 1 Corinthians 9:27 "But I discipline my body and keep it under control, lest after preaching to others I myself should be disqualified."

<u>Summary:</u> 1 Corinthians is one of two letters the Apostle Paul wrote to the group of believers in the Greek town of Corinth. In the book of Acts chapter 18 we learn that Paul visited the city of Corinth during his second missionary journey and was able to start a new church. We are told Paul stayed in Corinth for eighteen months. During that time he spent teaching and preaching God's Word to help the church mature and grow. It was this close relationship with the church that caused him to write two letters regarding his concern for spiritual and moral issues. When reading the early chapters of 1 Corinthians it doesn't take long to discover some of the problems they were having.

Quarrels, judging, divisions, lawsuits and unspeakable immorality are descriptive words for the issues going on, thus, this first letter of Paul's. Because this first letter didn't solve the problems a second letter was also written. Bottom line is, Paul says they need to get their act together.

Observation: Paul approaches the subject of "getting one's act together" by relating it to some very common sports activities with which the people would have been very familiar. In verse 24 he mentions running, in verse 25 he mentions sporting events, and in verse 26 he again mentions running and adds to it boxing. He is pointing out the fact that with all of these athletic events, in order to be successful, you have to take control of the situation, and in athletic events, that means taking control of your body, and literally making it do what you want it to do. When running make your body run in such a way that you will win. When competing in the games take control of your body in all ways, eat right, sleep enough and exercise. When boxing don't just throw wild punches, make sure you target your blows to a point for greatest impact. Verse 27 summarizes Paul's thoughts about what you have to do with your body in order to be a potential winner. You have to "discipline" your body. That means to take control of it, to make it your slave, to make it do what you want it to do. Only when you do this can you truly be a winner.

Application: So you want to win? You want to be able to bench press that additional weight? You want to win the local cross-fit competition? Then you've got to get control of your body. You've got to *discipline* it as the Apostle Paul puts it. Taking control of the body isn't easy. I can do great with my eating all day long and then blow the whole thing late at night when the ice cream starts calling out from the refrigerator. Major *discipline* has to happen in order for those early morning workouts to happen on a cold winter day in January. Remember, wining isn't easy, there are battles to fight, but they can be won. Now, don't forget the text for today. Paul is talking about the physical body, but mainly as an example. He was really targeting our moral, ethical and spiritual life. Are you winning in these areas of life? Make sure you *discipline* your body when it comes to the moral, ethical and spiritual parts of your life just as you *discipline* your body in the physical areas of life.

Day 16
Inner Beauty

Biblical Text: 1 Samuel 16:1-18

1) The Lord said to Samuel, "How long will you grieve over Saul, since I have rejected him from being king over Israel? Fill your horn with oil, and go. I will send you to Jesse the Bethlehemite, for I have provided for myself a king among his sons." 2) And Samuel said, "How can I go? If Saul hears it, he will kill me." And the Lord said, "Take a heifer with you and say, 'I have come to sacrifice to the Lord.' 3) And invite Jesse to the sacrifice, and I will show you what you shall do. And you shall anoint for me him whom I declare to you." 4) Samuel did what the Lord commanded and came to Bethlehem. The elders of the city came to meet him trembling and said, "Do you come peaceably?" 5) And he said, "Peaceably; I have come to sacrifice to the Lord. Consecrate yourselves, and come with me to the sacrifice." And he consecrated Jesse and his sons and invited them to the sacrifice.

6) When they came, he looked on Eliab and thought, "Surely the Lord's anointed is before him." 7) But the Lord said to Samuel, "Do not look on his appearance or on the height of his stature, because I have rejected him. For the Lord sees not as man sees: man looks on the outward appearance, but the Lord looks on the heart." 8) Then Jesse called Abinadab and made him pass before Samuel. And he said, "Neither has the Lord chosen this one." 9) Then Jesse made Shammah pass by. And he said,

"Neither has the Lord chosen this one." 10) And Jesse made seven of his sons pass before Samuel. And Samuel said to Jesse, "The Lord has not chosen these." 11) Then Samuel said to Jesse, "Are all your sons here?" And he said, "There remains yet the youngest, but behold, he is keeping the sheep." And Samuel said to Jesse, "Send and get him, for we will not sit down till he comes here." 12) And he sent and brought him in. Now he was ruddy and had beautiful eyes and was handsome. And the Lord said, "Arise anoint him, for this is he." 13) Then Samuel took the horn of oil and anointed him in the midst of his brothers. And the Spirit of the Lord rushed upon David from that day forward. And Samuel rose up and went to Ramah.

Theme Verse: 1 Samuel 16:7 "But the Lord said to Samuel, 'Do not look on his appearance or on the height of his stature, because I have rejected him. For the Lord sees not as man sees: man looks on the outward appearance, but the Lord looks on the heart.'"

Summary: Our reading for today brings us into the search for a new king for Israel. The present king, King Saul, has disobeyed God and is going to be replaced by someone who desires to please God in all things. The high priest and prophet, Samuel, has been sent on the search for the new king. God has led him to the home of a man named Jesse who has eight sons. God let Samuel know the new king would be chosen from these eight sons. Samuel assumed that because of the outward appearance of Eliab, he was the one chosen for the position of king. God reminded Samuel that as verse 7 states, "…For the Lord sees not as man sees: man looks on the outward appearance, but the Lord looks on the heart."

Observation: It doesn't take long as you grow up to realize outward appearance means a lot. In many cases, that's all that counts. The handsome or beautiful, and the well built or figured are the first to be chosen when choosing takes place. As a result, much time, effort and finances are given to crafting the best outward appearance one can obtain. I remember a chubby and homely little boy attending our son's seventh birthday party asking, "How can I be popular like you?" (Our seven year old was a cute athletic kid). At seven years old this boy already was dealing with the hard realities of getting ahead via outward appearance. But what about the heart, attitude, character, kindness, and compassion of someone? Doesn't this count at all?

Application: As you think about what kind of person you are, remember that the inner man, the heart, is very important to God. That's what he looks at when choosing individuals to serve him in special ways. However, this doesn't mean we don't therefore care how we look. The text of the day does comment on David's outward appearance in verse 12, "…Now he was ruddy and had beautiful eyes and was handsome," and verse 18 he's described as one "…who is skillful in playing, a man of valor, a man of war, prudent in speech, and a man of good presence…" Remember, it's not one to the exclusion of the other for even in these great descriptions of David it ends with "…and the Lord is with him" (vs. 18). Make sure you spend as much time beautifying the inner man as you do the outward man.

Day 17
Old Age Fitness

<u>Biblical Text:</u> Joshua 14:6-15

6) Then the people of Judah came to Joshua at Gilgal. And Caleb the son of Jephunneh the Kenizzite said to him, "You know what the Lord said to Moses the man of God in Kadesh-barnea concerning you and me. 7) I was forty years old when Moses the servant of the Lord sent me from Kadesh-barnea to spy out the land, and I brought him word again as it was in my heart. 8) But my brothers who went up with me made the heart of the people melt; yet I wholly followed the Lord my God. 9) And Moses swore on that day, saying, 'Surely the land on which your foot has trodden shall be an inheritance for you and your children forever, because you have wholly followed the Lord my God.' 10) And now, behold, the Lord has kept me alive, just as he said, these forty-five years since the time that the Lord spoke this word to Moses, while Israel walked in the wilderness. And now, behold, I am this day eighty-five years old. 11) I am still as strong today as I was in the day that Moses sent me; my strength now is as my strength was then, for war and for going and coming. 12) So now give me this hill country of which the Lord spoke on that day, for you heard on that day how the Anakim were there, with great fortified cities. It may be that the

Lord will be with me, and I shall drive them out just as the Lord said."

13) Then Joshua blessed him, and he gave Hebron to Caleb the son of Jephunneh for an inheritance. 14) Therefore Hebron became the inheritance of Caleb the son of Jephunneh the Kenizzite to this day, because he wholly followed the Lord, the God of Israel. 15) Now the name of Hebron formerly was Kiriatharba (Arba was the greatest man among the Anakim.) And the land had rest from war.

<u>Theme Verse:</u> Joshua 14:11 "I am still as strong today as I was in the day that Moses sent me; my strength now is as my strength was then, for war and for going and coming."

<u>Summary:</u> The book of Joshua records the historical events of the nation of Israel entering the land that God had promised to give them. The book of Exodus recounts how God rescues his people from slavery in the land of Egypt. The books of Leviticus, Numbers and Deuteronomy record the journey of God's people from Egypt to the promised land including their reluctance to enter the land promised them, an act of disobedience that lengthened their journey and entrance an additional forty years. Anyone over the age of twenty years at the time of this act of disobedience was not allowed to enter the promised land except for two men, Caleb and Joshua. They had both wanted to enter into the land of promise when they were originally supposed to. The forty-year delay was needed to give time for all of those over twenty

years of age to die, accept for Caleb and Joshua. Caleb, now eighty, has come to claim the promise.

Observation: Joshua chapter 14 addresses how some of the promised land was divided up, but its main focus is on the man named Caleb. At the time the nation originally came to the border of Israel Caleb was forty years old (vs. 7). We are also told that he, being one of the men sent to spy out the land, had trusted God for taking the land even though there were some big challenges ahead (vs. 7-8). Verse 9 tells us that because of Caleb's faithful trust in God he was to be given a certain part of the land as a reward. Our text today finds Caleb now eighty years old coming to claim what had been promised him. Joshua 14:11 tells us that Caleb had aged well and was very confident of his physical ability even now at eighty to claim the land God had promised him. We're not told why Caleb aged so well, but there does seem to be an indication that it was definitely related to his relationship with God. Verse 8 says, "…yet I wholly followed the Lord my God." Verse 14 repeats that same idea "…because he wholly followed the Lord, the God of Israel."

Application: When it comes to physical fitness the best thing we can remember is to work at staying fit all of our life thus enabling us to enjoy old age as much as our youth. It's not unusual when attending high school reunions to find that some of the most athletic men and women during high school years, now five, ten, fifteen and plus years later to be overweight with bulging guts and very unfit. What's the reason? Not maintaining fitness. The truth is, as we age, our fitness level declines. No matter how hard we work at trying to stay fit we just aren't going to maintain the same level of fitness we had in our twenty's, thirty's and even forty's when we reach the age of eighty. And though it may be a losing battle, doing nothing will definitely end life sooner. Making sure we regularly exercise and maintain as best a level of physical fitness all through our life is the best thing we can do. But don't forget what was said about Joshua in verses 8 and 14, "…he wholly followed the Lord…" God gave us his Word to both bless us and protect us. Thus as we strive to follow the Lord God there is no doubt our lives and the years we live will be better than they ever would be without the Lord.

Day 18
Standing Your Ground

<u>Biblical Text:</u> Daniel 1:1-16

1) In the third year of the reign of Jehoiakim king of Judah, Nebuchadnezzar king of Babylon came to Jerusalem and besieged it. 2) And the Lord gave Jehoiakim king of Judah into his hand, with some of the vessels of the house of God. And he brought them to the land of Shinar, to the house of his god, and placed the vessels in the treasury of his god. 3) Then the king commanded Ashpenaz, his chief eunuch, to bring some of the people of Israel, both of the royal family and of the nobility, 4) youths without blemish, of good appearance and skillful in all wisdom, endowed with knowledge, understanding, learning, and competent to stand in the king's palace, and to teach them the literature and language of the Chaldeans. 5) The king assigned them a daily portion of the food that the king ate, and of the wine that he drank. They were to be educated for three years, and at the end of that time they were to stand before the king. 6) Among these were Daniel, Hananiah, Mishael, and Azariah of the tribe of Judah. 7) And the chief of the eunuchs gave them names: Daniel he called Belteshazzar, Hananiah he called Shadrach, Mishael he called Meshach, and Azariah he called Abednego.

8) But Daniel resolved that he would not defile himself with the king's food, or with the wine that he drank. Therefore he asked the chief of the eunuchs to allow him not to defile himself. 9) And God gave Daniel favor and compassion in the sight of the chief of the eunuchs, 10) and the chief of the eunuchs said to Daniel, "I fear my lord the king, who assigned your food and your drink; for why should he see that you were in worse condition than the youths who are of your own age? So you would endanger my head with the king." 11) Then Daniel said to the steward whom the chief of the eunuchs had assigned over Daniel, Hananiah, Mishael, and Azariah, 12) "Test your servants for ten days; let us be given vegetables to eat and water to drink. 13) Then let our appearance and the appearance of the youths who eat the king's food be observed by you, and deal with your servants according to what you see." 14) So he listened to them in this matter, and tested them for ten days. 15) At the end of ten days it was seen that they were better in appearance and fatter in flesh than all the youths who ate the king's food. 16) So the steward took away their food and the wine they were to drink, and gave them vegetables.

Theme Verse: Daniel 1:8 "But Daniel resolved that he would not defile himself with the king's food, or with the wine that he drank. Therefore he asked the chief of the eunuchs to allow him not to defile himself."

Summary: Our text for today tells us the historical account of a young man named Daniel and three friends who are prisoners of war. In the ancient world it was not unusual for the victor to take the cream of the crop from the conquered and use their talents, abilities and experiences to advance his kingdom. Daniel and his three friends are in this group. They are described as physically fit, good looking, intelligent and poised. But even with these outstanding characteristics the King of Babylon needed to help them shed any vestige of the culture and life they had come from and be indoctrinated into being Babylonians, thus the instruction to the overseer to educate them, give them the best of the kingdom and give them new names.

Observation: At first one might think that the issue had to do with them being vegetarians. And since they ended up looking better after ten days on such a diet compared to those who ate the king's food there is a strong argument for such a diet. However, deeper truths are being taught. The main issue has to do with the battle to compromise. Daniel and his friends had a commitment to their God and they had been trained in the things that pleased God. Their faith, what we know of today as Judaism, did not teach that God is pleased with vegetarians. But he is not displeased with them either. The greater issue here was giving up the truths they knew for the false things the Babylonians wanted to give them.

Application: One of the biggest battles facing the person who desires to be fit is the battle of compromise. As you research fitness you begin to understand things you need to do to become fit. So based on this information you lay out an eating plan and an exercise plan. Then you go out and spend money on a gym membership or equipment to set up a home gym. You start with great intentions with eating right and exercising according to the plan and you begin to feel great about yourself. What happens? The battle for compromise begins to rage. You are late for a meeting and so you decide to get some fast food. One time won't hurt. The alarm clock goes off, but since it was a late night you decide fifteen more minutes in bed will do you better than pumping iron. How do you win this battle? Be a Daniel, "But Daniel resolved…" (vs. 8). Commit yourself to your plan and no matter what, don't compromise. And just as you are uncompromising with your physical fitness plan be uncompromising with your spiritual fitness plan. Do you have a plan to become spiritually fit? If not, seek out someone how can help you develop one.

Obedience

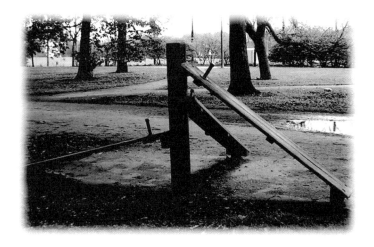

Day 19
Physical Health

Biblical Text: Proverbs 3:5-8

> 5) Trust in the Lord with all your heart,
>   and do not lean on your own
>   understanding.
> 6) In all your ways acknowledge him,
>   and he will make straight your paths.
> 7) Be not wise in your own eyes;
>   fear the Lord, and turn away from
>   evil.
> 8) It will be healing to your flesh
>   and refreshment to your bones.

Theme Verse: Proverbs 3:7-8
> Be not wise in your own eyes;
>   fear the Lord, and turn away from
>   evil.
> It will be healing to your flesh
>   and refreshment to your bones.

Summary: The book of Proverbs was written by a man named Solomon. He was king over Israel from 992 to 961 B.C. He was known throughout the ancient world as the wisest man on the face of the earth. His wisdom was so renown that people travelled from great distances to learn from him. Why was Solomon so wise? Because, at the beginning of his reign, he asked God to give him wisdom. His request is recorded for us in 1 Kings 3:9, "Give your servant, therefore, an understanding mind to govern your people, that I may discern between good and evil, for who is able to govern this your great people?" He knew he had a difficult task before him and the only way to accomplish it was to be given wisdom from the one who is wisdom, God. Solomon gives us excellent counsel on all the issues of life, but he begins by making sure we understand that wise decisions and wise living have their beginning in a right relationship with God. Find his first words of counsel for us in Proverbs 1:7, "The fear of the Lord is the beginning of knowledge…"

Observation: It's interesting to note the breadth of subjects Solomon's wisdom covers. It isn't just spiritual areas like in Proverbs 15:9, "The way of the wicked is an abomination to the Lord, but he loves him who pursues righteousness." It isn't just emotional areas like in Proverbs 15:13, "A glad heart makes a cheerful face, but by sorrow of heart the spirit is crushed." It isn't just relational areas like in Proverbs 15:1, "A soft answer turns away wrath, but a harsh word stirs up anger." His wisdom even covers physical areas of our life as stated in our text today, Proverbs 3:8, "It will be healing to your flesh and refreshment to your bones."

Application: Bookstores and magazine racks are filled with man's wisdom on the subject of physical fitness and health. Do you want to bulk up your muscles? Then do heavy weights with fewer reps. If you want your muscles to be well defined and able to endure, then do less weight and more reps. Do you want to lose weight? Take in fewer calories than calories expended in the day. Do you want to stave off osteoporosis? Then make sure you are doing some kind of strength training as it increases bone density. These things are man's wisdom. But what does the all-wise God, the creator of our bodies say about physical health? His maintenance manual (the Bible) for his created creatures says that physical health and strong bones actually come from trusting in God, seeking his way in all things and finally, turning away from evil. Having tried all of man's ideas on physical fitness, don't you think it's about time to try using God's wisdom?

Day 20
Strong But Dumb

Biblical Text: Judges 16:4-22

4) After this he loved a woman in the Valley of Sorek, whose name was Delilah. 5) And the lords of the Philistines came up to her and said to her, "Seduce him, and see where his great strength lies, and by what means we may overpower him, that we may bind him to humble him. And we will each give you 1,100 pieces of silver." 6) So Delilah said to Samson, "Please tell me where your great strength lies, and how you might be bound, that one could subdue you."

7) Samson said to her, "If they bind me with seven fresh bowstrings that have not been dried, then I shall become weak and be like any other man." 8) Then the lords of the Philistines brought up to her seven fresh bowstrings that had not been dried, and she bound him with them. 9) Now she had men lying in ambush in an inner chamber. And she said to him, "The Philistines are upon you, Samson!" But he snapped the bowstrings, as a thread of flax snaps when it touches the fire. So the secret of his strength was not known.

10) Then Delilah said to Samson, "Behold, you have mocked me and told me lies. Please tell me how you might be bound." 11) And he said to her, "If they bind me with new ropes that have not been used, then I shall

become weak and be like any other man." 12) So Delilah took new ropes and bound him with them and said to him, "The Philistines are upon you, Samson!" And the men lying in ambush were in an inner chamber But he snapped the ropes off his arms like a thread.

13) Then Delilah said to Samson, "Until now you have mocked me and told me lies. Tell me how you might be bound." And he said to her, "If you weave the seven locks of my head with the web and fasten it tight with the pin, then I shall become weak and be like any other man." 14) So while he slept, Delilah took the seven locks of his head and wove them into the web. And she made them tight with the pin and said to him, "The Philistines are upon you, Samson!" But he awoke from his sleep and pulled away the pin, the loom, and the web.

15) And she said to him, "How can you say, 'I love you,' when your heart is not with me? You have mocked me these three times, and you have not told me where your great strength lies." 16) And when she pressed him hard with her words day after day, and urged him, his soul was vexed to death. 17) And he told her all his heart, and said to her, "A razor has never come upon my head, for I have been a Nazirite to God from my mother's womb. If my head is shaved, then my strength will leave me, and I shall become weak and be like any other man."

18) When Delilah saw that he had told her all his heart, she sent and called the lords of

the Philistines, saying, "Come up again, for he has told me all his heart." Then the lords of the Philistines came up to her and brought the money in their hands. 19) She made him sleep on her knees. And she called a man and had him shave off the seven locks of his head. Then she began to torment him, and his strength left him. 20) And she said, "The Philistines are upon you, Samson!" And he awoke from his sleep and said, "I will go out as at other times and shake myself free." But he did not know that the Lord had left him. 21) And the Philistines seized him and gouged out his eyes and brought him down to Gaza and bound him with bronze shackles. And he ground at the mill in the prison. 22) But the hair of his head began to grow again after it had been shaved.

Theme Verse: Judges 16:20 "And she said, 'The Philistines are upon you, Samson!' And he awoke from his sleep and said, 'I will go out as at other times and shake myself free.' But he did not know that the Lord had left him."

Summary: A full account of Samson's life is found in Judges 13:1-16:31. His biography presents him as specially appointed by God to be a rescuer of the Israelites. Thus God endowed him with extraordinary physical strength to do his work. We might say that he is the biblical equivalent of a modern day body builder. We know that Samson was strong, because of the things he did. He killed a lion with his bare hands; he won a fight with the odds being thirty to one; he caught 300 foxes and tied their tails together; he broke ropes that bound him; he carried a city gate to the top of a hill. There seems to be no end to his feats of strength. But even the strongest have weaknesses, and his was a weakness for women. At first we might think that it was this weakness which led to his defeat, but the truth is that his defeat came because he didn't acknowledge God as the giver of his strength and live in obedience to him.

Observation: Having spent hours, days, weeks, months, and possibly years pumping iron in a gym it is easy for you to think that your strength is all because of your effort. No doubt that was what happened to Samson. Having accomplished multiple acts of strength, his understanding of where his strength came from became clouded. It became so clouded that he forgot that God had prepared him to serve him in a special way. The result was that he thought he could accomplish God's work without him. It led even to the point at which he thought he could be disobedient to God's Word and, living in sin, still do the work of God. How foolish Samson was! You can't accomplish God's work without him.

Application: Are you thinking like Samson? Impressed with your strength and abilities? Are you thinking that you are who you are and what you are as a result of your own efforts? Are there sin issues in your life that you are not dealing with because you think trying to serve God just doesn't matter? Next time you exercise, stop and take a moment to thank God for making you who you are, and say, "Search me, O God, and know my heart! Try me and know my thoughts! And see if there be any grievous way in me, and lead me in the way everlasting!" (Psalm 139:23-24). There is nothing worse than trying to serve God in your own strength, without him.

Day 21
Fight Your Way Out

<u>Biblical Text:</u> Jeremiah 9:23-24

> 23) Thus says the Lord: "Let not the wise man boast in his wisdom, let not the mighty man boast in his might, let not the rich man boast in his riches, 24) but let him who boasts boast in this, that he understands and knows me, that I am the Lord who practices steadfast love, justice, and righteousness in the earth. For in these things I delight, declares the Lord."

<u>Theme Verse:</u> Jeremiah 9:23 "Thus says the Lord: 'Let not the wise man boast in his wisdom, let not the might man boast in his might, let not the rich man boast in his riches,'"

<u>Summary:</u> In the nation of Judah, lived God's chosen people. As his people they were supposed to honor God with their allegiance and obedience to him. But they neither gave him their allegiance nor obeyed him. As a result God sent his prophet, Jeremiah, to warn them of God's coming judgment. You can read about his charge against them and the resulting punishment in Jeremiah 9:12-16. Even with the warning from the prophet, the people of Judah did not turn back to God. Instead they trumpeted their own ability to deal with the trouble that was going to come upon them. Verse 23 tells us they thought they were wise enough, mighty enough and rich enough that no matter what troubles

came their way they could handle it. They thought very highly of themselves.

Observation: Our culture believes much the same way the ancient people of Judah believed. If you have wisdom, might and riches you can solve any problem that comes your way. So we get education to gain wisdom; we go to the gym to get might; we go to the stock market to get rich. With these things we can think our way out, fight our way out, or buy our way out of any problem that comes our way.

Application: Can you see how this happens? Work on widening your shoulders and pumping up the biceps and no one is going to bother you. I remember years ago, one of the early body builders of our age advertising his exercise program in comic books. The ad showed a bully on a beach kicking sand in the face of a scrawny young man. If you sent for the muscle-building program you would never have to let bullies kick sand in your face again. But all muscle does when trying to solve problems is generally create a bigger fight. Verse 24 of our text says the thing we should boast in is our relationship with God. The reason for this is that it changes the inside of man, the heart, the thinking. It is these changes and walking in obedience to God that is going to address the major problems that come your way, not brain, brawn or a big bundle.

Day 22
Fit to Serve

Biblical Text: Acts 8:26-40

26) Now an angel of the Lord said to Philip, "Rise and go toward the south to the road that goes down from Jerusalem to Gaza." This is a desert place. 27) And he rose and went. And there was an Ethiopian, a eunuch, a court official of Candace, queen of the Ethiopians, who was in charge of all her treasure. He had come to Jerusalem to worship 28) and was returning, seated in his chariot, and he was reading the prophet Isaiah. 29) And the Spirit said to Philip, "Go over and join this chariot." 30) So Philip ran to him and heard him reading Isaiah the prophet and asked, "Do you understand what you are reading?" 31) And he said, "How can I, unless someone guides me?" And he invited Philip to come up and sit with him. 32) Now the passage of the Scripture that he was reading was this:

Like a sheep he was led to the slaughter
and like a lamb before its shearer is silent,
so he opens not his mouth.
33)   In his humiliation justice was denied him.

Who can describe his generation?
For his life is taken away from the
earth."

34) And the eunuch said to Philip, "About whom, I ask you, does the prophet say this, about himself or about someone else?" 35) Then Philip opened his mouth, and beginning with this Scripture he told him the good news about Jesus. 36) And as they were going along the road they came to some water, and the eunuch said, "See, here is water! What prevents me from being baptized?" 38) And he commanded the chariot to stop, and they both went down into the water, Philip and the eunuch, and he baptized him. 39) And when they came up out of the water, the Spirit of the Lord carried Philip away, and the eunuch saw him no more, and went on his way rejoicing. 40) But Philip found himself at Azotus, and as he passed through he preached the gospel to all the towns until he came to Caesarea.

Theme Verse: Acts 8:30 "So Philip ran to him and heard him reading Isaiah the prophet and asked, 'Do you understand what you are reading?'"

Summary: Acts 8:26-40 gives the historical account of a high government official finding Jesus Christ as Savior. We know little about him other than that he is a eunuch and is in charge of the treasure that belongs to an Ethiopian queen named Candace. But, most important, he is a seeker after God. In this account we find him reading an Old Testament prophecy about the crucifixion of Jesus Christ. Not understanding what he is reading, he realizes that he needs someone to explain the prophecy. In response to this seeker's need, God directs a man named Philip to go and help him. Because Philip is obedient to God, this prominent government official becomes a follower of Jesus Christ. It is believed that, following his conversion, he returned to Ethiopia and shared the "Good News," and what we know today as the Orthodox Church began.

Observation: Think about the physical challenge that confronted Philip in order to make him obedient to God's direction. He had to travel from the city of Samaria (Acts 8:4) to an unspecified location on the road from Jerusalem to Gaza, a distance of unknown miles. It would be unusual if this had not been done on foot. Then at the end of the journey, Philip had to run fast enough to catch up with a moving chariot. We don't know if Philip was a track star in his local school or not, but we do know that he was fit enough to walk many miles and end the journey with a sprint. It can be truly said that Philip was physically fit enough to accomplish the special task God had for him.

Application: The Bible is very clear that God has work for all of us to accomplish for him. In general, we know that it is important to be spiritually prepared and biblically knowledgeable, so that we can accomplish the work God gives us. But, when was the last time you asked yourself if your fitness level was sufficient to accomplish the work God has for you? It is very important that our fitness level does not stand in the way of serving God. Work at getting fit, or staying fit, so you can do the special work that God has for you.

Day 23
Strength Training

Biblical Text: 2 Timothy 2:1-13

1) You then, my child, be strengthened by the grace that is in Christ Jesus, 2) and what you have heard from me in the presence of many witnesses entrust to faithful men who will be able to teach others also. 3) Share in suffering as a good soldier of Christ Jesus. 4) No soldier gets entangled in civilian pursuits, since his aim is to please the one who enlisted him. 5) An athlete is not crowned unless he competes according to the rules. 6) It is the hard-working farmer who ought to have the first share of the crops. 7) Think over what I say, for the Lord will give you understanding in everything.

8) Remember Jesus Christ, risen from the dead, the offspring of David, as preached in my gospel, 9) for which I am suffering, bound with chains as a criminal. But the word of God is not bound! Therefore I endure everything for the sake of the elect, that they also may obtain the salvation that is in Christ Jesus with eternal glory. 11) The saying is trustworthy, for:

> If we have died with him, we will also
> live with him;
> 12) if we endure, we will also reign with
> him;
> if we deny him, he also will deny us;

13)   if we are faithless, he remains
                    faithful--
for he cannot deny himself.

Theme Verse: 2 Timothy 2:5 "An athlete is not crowned unless he competes according to the rules."

Summary: 2 Timothy is the second of two letters that the Apostle Paul wrote to a young man named Timothy. We learn in verses 3 and 4 of the first letter that Timothy had been left by Paul in the city of Ephesus to deal with problems in the church, the teaching of false and unimportant things. In 4:12 of this first letter we also learn Timothy is young and in the Greek culture of that time this would not have helped his level of authority to do the work Paul asks of him. Both of Paul's letters to Timothy give him guidance in a number of areas of church structure, leadership and living a life for Christ. Timothy needed to be encouraged to press on and complete the tasks Paul left him to do. Thus the words in 2 Timothy 2:1, "...be strengthened..."

Observation: Paul tells Timothy how he can be strong. He gives three different examples that highlight certain elements essential for strength. First is the soldier who doesn't get involved in things pertaining to his goal. This could be called "focus." Second is the athlete who is only going to win if he follows the rules. This could be called "following the plan." Third is the farmer who displays the essentials of hard work. This is called "hard work." Paul is telling Timothy that the strength he needs to complete the task for which he's been left in Ephesus is to "stay focused" on what he's suppose to do; "stay with the plan" they developed; and "work hard" at both. These three simple truths will help him stay strong; however, notice that ultimately these are anchored in Christ Jesus.

Application: While Paul is talking about being strong in the area of leadership, these three elements are also essential for physical strength. And in the end good leadership requires being healthy which requires some physical strength. Think how important "focus" is when it comes to strength training. Unless you stay focused on the task all kinds of things are going to keep you from getting to the gym to hit the weights. Being too tired, having too much to do, preferring to do something else never leads to the physical strength you want. How about following the rules or "staying with the plan?" Muscles only get stronger and grow if the form of a particular exercise is followed. And if you've got a plan to help you move ahead, deviation from the plan doesn't bring you the success you want. "Hard work?" Nothing needs to be said on this other than the reminder that growing in physical strength demands hard work. But what good is physical strength if not applied to essential things of life? Just being strong for the purpose of being strong makes no sense; it's a worthless effort. Physical strength needs to be applied to something. How about using it to help you be the best leader you can be? How about using it to serve Jesus Christ and the purposes He has for you. When anchored in Jesus "staying focused," "staying with the plan" and "working hard" all make sense and will make service and leadership for Jesus Christ much easier.

Day 24
Growing Old

Biblical Text: 2 Corinthians 4:16-5:10

4:16) So we do not lose heart. Though our outer nature is wasting away, our inner nature is being renewed day by day.17) For this slight momentary affliction is preparing for us an eternal weight of glory beyond all comparison, 18) as we look not to the things that are seen but to the things that are unseen. For the things that are seen are transient, but the things that are unseen are eternal.

5:1) For we know that if the tent, which is our earthly home is destroyed, we have a building from God, a house not made with hands, eternal in the heavens. 2) For in this tent we groan, longing to put on our heavenly dwelling, 3) if indeed by putting it on we may not be found naked. 4) For while we are still in this tent, we groan, being burdened - not that we would be unclothed, but that we would be further clothed, so that what is mortal may be swallowed up by life. 5) He who has prepared us for this very thing is God, who has given us the Spirit as a guarantee.

6) So we are always of good courage. We know that while we are at home in the body we are away from the Lord, 7) for we walk by faith, not by sight. 8) Yes, we are of good courage, and we would rather be away from the body and at home with the Lord. 9)

So whether we are at home or away, we make it our aim to please him. 10) For we must all appear before the judgment seat of Christ, so that each one may receive what is due for what he has done in the body; whether good or evil.

Theme Verse: 2 Corinthians 4:16 "So we do not lose heart. Though our outer nature is wasting away, our inner nature is being renewed day by day."

Summary: The book of 2 Corinthians is the second of two letters the Apostle Paul wrote to the community of believers in the city of Corinth, Greece. Both letters address theological, ethical and moral issues with which the people were struggling. Because of his past relationship with the people and his continued love for them he writes words of instruction, challenge and correction calling them to be people of God as described in 2 Corinthians 5:17, "Therefore, if anyone is in Christ, he is a new creation. The old has passed away; behold, the new has come." Throughout Paul's two letters he also has to address the questioning of his authority. This, of course, causes great challenge to him, just one of many things that causes him challenges in life. Our section of reading today takes up the theme of challenges in life that confront Paul and us.

Observation: In our reading of today, Paul raises the challenge each one of us faces, troubles in life and the body growing old. Notice the words he uses to describe our situation, "our outer self is wasting away," "light momentary affliction," "the tent that is our earthly home is destroyed," "in this tent we groan," "we groan, being burdened." Troubles in life and growing old have been a challenge to people throughout history and has led in the effort to extend life. Ponce de Leon, the Spanish explorer who discovered Florida in 1513 was actually seeking to find the mythical fountain of youth heard of in Indian legends. The recent Disney movie called "Tangled," the fairytale story of Rapunzel, presented the desire of the wicked woman to stay young. Botox and cryogenics are all man's efforts to confront the results of aging. But as the bumper sticker says "Eat Healthy, Exercise Regularly, Die Anyway." The truth is, no matter what we do, we age and die. This is why it's important to focus on the contrasting theme found in our text of today, "our inner self is being renewed day by day," "an eternal weight of glory beyond all comparison," "we have a building from God, a house not made with hands, eternal in the heavens," "longing to put on our heavenly dwelling;" But notice the promise of God in our reading, "we have a building from God," "eternal in the heavens." These are wonderful promises and we know they are true because as God said, he "gave to us the Spirit as a pledge."

Application: So if growing old and the decaying of my body is certain, why give any effort to taking care of my body by faithfully exercising and eating right? The answer for us is found in 5:9 "So whether we are at home or away, we make it our aim to please him." I take care of my body so that I can do all that God has called me to do. He has certain tasks for me to do while here on earth and I want to be as healthy and able to do them as I can. I truly want to please him on earth as long as I can. Furthermore even though body decay and death is certain I don't have to live in fear of death. Twice in these verses Paul speaks of "good courage." I press ahead in the earthly seen life because I have the promise of a present unseen life that is in heaven and eternal. So remain faithful to fitness. You can't stop body decay or aging but you can slow it up. In this earthly life and earthly body be pleasing to God.

Day 25
Personal Fitness Trainer

Biblical Text: Acts 18:24-28

24) Now a Jew named Apollos, a native of Alexandria, came to Ephesus. He was an eloquent man, competent in the Scriptures. 25) He had been instructed in the way of the Lord. And being fervent in spirit, he spoke and taught accurately the things concerning Jesus, though he knew only the baptism of John. 26) He began to speak boldly in the synagogue, but when Priscilla and Aquila heard him, they took him and explained to him the way of God more accurately. 27) And when he wished to cross to Achaia, the brothers encouraged him and wrote to the disciples to welcome him. When he arrived, he greatly helped those who through grace had believed, 28) for he powerfully refuted the Jews in public, showing by the Scriptures that the Christ was Jesus.

Theme Verse: Acts 18:28 "for he powerfully refuted the Jews in public, showing by the Scriptures that the Christ was Jesus."

Summary: The New Testament section of the Bible begins with what are called the Gospels: Matthew, Mark, Luke and John. This is the historical account of God coming in the flesh, living among us as the person we know named Jesus, and preaching "Good News" to us. The "Good News" is that Jesus was going to take care of our sin problem. The book of Acts continues the historical narrative by recording how the "Good News" impacted people of the world and how God lives in our presence through the Holy Spirit. Acts 18 introduces us to a follower of Jesus named Apollos. As we read about his life we learn how important it is to know as much as we can about Jesus. We also learn how others who are stronger in their understanding of Jesus can help us grow in our faith. This is called "discipling."

Observation: One of the things I first note about the man named Apollos is that he was "competent in the Scriptures" (vs. 24). This means he knew them well. We also learn that he was allowing the Holy Spirit, who dwelt in him, to guide the work he was doing. But it's clear from the text he still had some things to learn, as he only knew the account of Jesus up to a certain point. Introduced into the story are a married couple named Priscilla and Aquila who after hearing his preaching, boldly take him aside and begin to teach him. This is called discipling. As a result of their discipling, Apollos becomes even more capable in proclaiming the truth about Jesus. This is not too dissimilar to fitness training. I've done some reading, Google searches and watched others in gyms as they exercise. As a result feel like I have a fairly good handle on what I think I need to do to get fit, having more strength and endurance. I love when I come to a weight machine and note that I can add weight to the machine and outdo the woman or better yet, the man who used the machine prior to me. But admittedly I don't know it all so could and should use the help of others who know more about fitness than I.

Application: How would you evaluate your understanding of fitness? Do you think you know it all? Do you possibly think, "I don't need anyone's help?" The worse place one can be is living in the lie of arrogance and thinking we know it all. I'm always amazed when watching sporting events on television that the best gymnasts, ice skaters, and tennis players still have coaches and trainers. Why is that? It's because they don't live a life of arrogance thinking they know it all. They know they can always improve in their sport. Not moving ahead to the level you'd like in fitness? Be willing to seek out some help, get some advice. Maybe take a few sessions from a personal fitness trainer; maybe take a class. How's your spiritual fitness? Do you think you know it all; everything there is to know about the scriptures. Make sure you spend time learning from someone else whose walk with Christ has been longer than yours and grown deeper than you. So just as you might seek out a personal fitness trainer or class for your physical life, think seriously about finding someone to disciple you or get involved in a Bible study where you can learn more about walking with Christ.

Self-Reflection

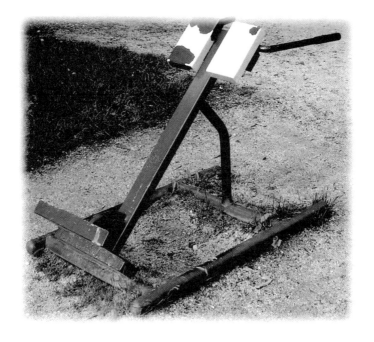

Day 26
God Did Well When He Made You

<u>Biblical Text:</u> Psalm 139:1-24

To The Choirmaster. A Psalm of David.

1) O Lord, you have searched me and
   known me!
2) You know when I sit down and when I
   rise up;
   you discern my thoughts from afar.
3) You search out my path and my lying
   down
   and are acquainted with all my ways.
4) Even before a word is on my tongue,
   behold, O Lord, you know it
   altogether.
5) You hem me in, behind and before,
   and lay your hand upon me.
6) Such knowledge is too wonderful
   for me;
   it is high; I cannot attain it.

7) Where shall I go from your Spirit?
   Or where shall I flee from your
   presence?
8) If I ascend to heaven, you are there!
   If I make my bed in Sheol, you are
   there!
9) If I take the wings of the morning
   and dwell in the uttermost parts of the
   sea,

10) even there your hand shall lead me,
    and your right hand shall hold me.
11) If I say, "Surely the darkness shall
      cover me,
  and the light about me be night,"
12) even the darkness is not dark to you;
    the night is bright as the day;
    for darkness is as light with you.

13) For you formed my inward parts;
    you knitted me together in my
      mother's womb.
14) I praise you, for I am fearfully and
    wonderfully made.
  Wonderful are your works;
    my soul knows it very well.
15) My frame was not hidden from you,
  when I was being made in secret,
    intricately woven in the depths of the
      earth.
16) Your eyes saw my uniformed substance;
  in your book were written, every one of
      them,
    the days that were formed for me,
    when as yet there were none of them.

17) How precious to me are your thoughts,
    O God!
  How vast is the sum of them!
18) If I would count them, they are more
      than the sand.
  I awake, and I am still with you.

19) Oh that you would slay the wicked,
O God!
O men of blood, depart from me!
20) They speak against you with malicious
intent;
your enemies take your name in vain!
21) Do I not hate those who hate you,
O Lord?
And do I not loathe those who rise up
against you?
22) I hate them with complete hatred;
I count them my enemies.

23) Search me, O God, and know my heart!
Try me and know my thoughts!
24) And see if there be any grievous way
in me,
and lead me in the way everlasting!

Theme Verse: Psalm 139:13
"For you formed my inward parts;
you knitted me together in my
mother's womb."

Summary: King David writes a wonderful Psalm about God's omnipresence and omniscience. The word "omnipresence" describes how God is everywhere, and the word "omniscience" describes how God knows everything. He teaches these truths about God by describing all the places God is, and all the things God knows. The encouragement to me is that wherever I am, God is there with me. Whether I'm having the greatest day, "If I ascend to heaven…" (vs.

8), or the worst day of my life "…If I make my bed in Sheol…" (vs. 8), God is right there with me "…you are there!" (vs. 8). It also teaches that God knows everything. Again, this is very encouraging, but it can also be disconcerting. Does he really know what I'm thinking?

Observation: It's important to note that God's omnipresence and omniscience come into play with what I look like. Verses 13 through 16 clearly indicate that I look like I do because this is what God wanted. In his greatness, he chose to make me tall or short, big or small nosed, or of a particular ethnicity; and though we may not understand, he planned even a deformity for his purposes.

Application: So what do we do with how we look? Verse 14 says, "I praise you, for I am fearfully and wonderfully made…" So the things that can't be changed without artificial means leave alone unless health reasons demand change and thank God for them. Leave the nose the size it is. Forget Botox treatments, and enjoy aging. But the things that can be changed with fitness, feel free to do so. You are not overweight because God did it to you. You just made too many trips to the refrigerator and sat around too much. Change the things that can be naturally changed; leave the things that can't be naturally changed. So hit the road, pool, treadmill, and weights, and watch what you eat. And thank God daily for how you look, for in his omniscience you look just like he wants you to look.

Day 27
Likeable

<u>Biblical Text:</u> Proverbs 3:1-8

1) My son, do not forget my teaching,
    but let your heart keep my
        commandments,
2) for length of days and years of life
    are peace they will add to you.
3) Let not steadfast love and faithfulness
        forsake you;
    bind them around your neck;
    write them on the tablet of your heart.
4) So you will find favor and good success
    in the sight of God and man.

5) Trust in the Lord with all your heart,
    and do not lean on your own
        understanding.
6) In all your ways acknowledge him,
    and he will make straight your paths.
7) Be not wise in your own eyes;
    fear the Lord, and turn away from
        evil.
8) It will be healing to your flesh
    and refreshment to your bones.

<u>Theme Verse:</u> Proverbs 3:4
    "So you will find favor and good success
        in the sight of God and man."

Summary: Today we find ourselves in a book of the Bible called wisdom literature. The book teaches us about wisdom, what it is, its importance, how to gain it and its end result. Much of this is taught by contrasting it with foolishness. Today's reading focuses on the rewards of wisdom. Verses 1 and 2 teach us that in general if you live your life according to the Bible you will experience a peaceful and long life. Verses 3 and 4 teach us that if we are kind and truthful we will have a good reputation. Verses 5 thru 7 teach us that when Jesus Christ is our Lord, allowing him to rule our life instead of ourselves, our whole physical form and make-up will generally be in good health.

Observation: When it comes to being well respected by others, what a sharp contrast the book of Proverbs is compared to the ways of the world. The world says exercise and train hard. You'll impress people by how you look, you'll live longer and, if you really do well, you might even get in the big league of sports and gain fame and fortune. So do whatever it takes. Do what is best for YOU and you will have great rewards. By contrast, Proverbs says think of others and let Christ rule and tell you what's best.

Application: It is so easy when striving after fitness to focus totally on self and what others say and think about how you look. It's easy to forget what life is really about. That's why the text reminds us in verse 1 "…do not forget…" and in verse 3 "Let not steadfast love and faithfulness forsake you;…" Be fit, but ever keeping the teachings of scripture at the forefront of our life will cause people to want to be with us.

Day 28
Taking Care of the Garden

Biblical Text: Genesis 2:10-17

10) A river flowed out of Eden to water the garden, and there it divided and became four rivers. 11) The name of the first is the Pishon. It is the one that flowed around the whole land of Havilah, where there is gold. 12) And the gold of that land is good; bdellium and onyx stone are there. 13) The name of the second river is the Gihon. It is the one that flowed around the whole land of Cush. 14) And the name of the third river is the Tigris, which flows east of Assyria. And the fourth river is the Euphrates.

15) The Lord God took the man and put him in the garden of Eden to work it and keep it. 16) And the Lord God commanded the man, saying, "You may surely eat of every tree of the garden, 17) but of the tree of the knowledge of good and evil you shall not eat, for in the day that you eat of it you shall surely die."

Theme Verse: Genesis 2:15 "The Lord God took the man and put him in the garden of Eden to work it and keep it.

Summary: The first book of the Bible, the book of Genesis, begins with stating two facts: 1) There is a God, and 2) God created everything. It's interesting that the Bible makes no arguments to back up these statements. The statements stand alone as truth. Whether you agree with these declarative statements or not, it's important to note that over and over again everything he creates is described as "good." When he finally creates man and woman, he is so impressed with his work that he declares it to be "very good." The verses of today seem to indicate that since God's creative work is "good," he wanted the man he created to take care of it. He had two tasks: to work it and to keep it. The activity of working the soil, also known as cultivating or tilling the soil, would help the garden grow and the activity of keeping it would help the garden endure or last.

Observation: It's interesting to note that when it comes to instructions regarding the care of God's creation the only thing that is mentioned is care for the garden. But if special care was to be given to the garden, which God called "good," can we not infer that God would also want the man and woman to take care of their bodies since they too are his creation? After all, they were described as "very good." So if that which was called "good" was to be worked and kept, should not that which was called "very good" also be worked (cultivated) and kept?

Application: How is it we work and keep our bodies, the two activities given by God to take care of his other acts of creation? Since working ground is an activity that causes crops to grow, mature and be healthy, we can assume the working of the human body would need activities to do these very things. Thus the importance of doing activities that help the body grow, mature and be healthy. This would include such things as strength training, cardio training, good eating habits, and adequate amounts of sleep. All of these things are essential for a body, created by God to be healthy. The other term used for the care of the garden was "keep." This word actually means to "protect from harm." It doesn't take one any length of time to make a list of things that harm one's health. A small sample would be hours of sitting at the computer or in front of the TV, poor eating habits, stress, steroids and other drugs. If you are going to guard God's creation you need to protect it from these types of things. One of the best things you can do to keep at the two tasks God has given you to care for his creation is to remember what he thinks about you. He says, you are "very good." Let's have the same attitude about our bodies as God does.

Day 29
Building Maintenance

<u>Biblical Text:</u> 1 Corinthians 6:12-20

12) "All things are lawful for me," but not all things are helpful. "All things are lawful for me," but I will not be enslaved by anything. 13) "Food is meant for the stomach and the stomach for food"-and God will destroy both one and the other. The body is not meant for sexual immorality, but for the Lord, and the Lord for the body. 14) And God raised the Lord and will also raise us up by his power. 15) Do you not know that your bodies are members of Christ? Shall I then take the members of Christ and make them members of a prostitute? Never! 16) Or do you not know that he who is joined to a prostitute becomes one body with her? For, as it is written, "The two will become one flesh." 17) But he who is joined to the Lord becomes one spirit with him. 18) Flee from sexual immorality. Every other sin a person commits is outside the body, but the sexually immoral person sins against his own body. 19) Or do you not know that your body is a temple of the Holy Spirit within you, whom you have from God? You are not your own, 20) for you were bought with a price. So glorify God in your body.

<u>Theme Verse:</u> 1 Corinthians 6:19 "Or do you not know that your body is a temple of the Holy Spirit within

you, whom you have from God? You are not your own."

Summary: God's Word makes an amazing statement. It declares that our bodies are the building in which God lives. When we are converted, the third person of the triune Godhead, known as the Holy Spirit, takes up residence in our physical bodies. It helps to understand this when we remember that, in the Old Testament, God's Spirit first dwelt in a tent that traveled with the children of Israel on their journey from Egypt to Israel, and then in the Jerusalem temple that King Solomon built. Each of these residences was built at great cost, using the finest of products. Following their construction, they were maintained adhering to very strict guidelines. Thus this Bible passage is very concerned about how we maintain our physical bodies, since they have been constructed (bought, vs. 20) at a great cost. That cost was the death and shedding of Jesus Christ's blood on the cross, taking the punishment that we should receive for our sins.

Observation: Our text points out some interesting things about how we treat our bodies. There are two categories dealt with: 1) things we put into our bodies; and 2) things we do with our bodies. On the subject of what we put into our bodies, most people who have walked with Christ for years would agree that such things as smoking and drugs damage the body. But what about donuts, pizza and potato chips? Don't such diets lead to overweight, and overweight to heart issues or adult onset diabetes? On the subject of "shacking up" with a prostitute (vs. 16), there would probably be no argument that you should not do that to your body. But what about sitting, hour after hour, in front of the TV set or computer? Such inactivity leads to the same thing as a bad diet. The Holy Spirit's residence, your physical body, needs to be well maintained.

Summary: If you have been converted to Jesus Christ, then the Holy Spirit dwells in you. It costs Jesus Christ his life to make this temple for the Holy Spirit. It is now your responsibility to maintain it. Does a diet of donuts, pizza, and such foods help maintain the temple? Does a life of inactivity, or hours spent in front of the computer and TV, maintain the temple? Verse 12 puts it clearly: "…I will not be enslaved by anything," and that includes food or technology. Review your present temple maintenance, and make the necessary changes.

Day 30
Finding Strength in Weakness

Biblical Text: 2 Corinthians 12:7-10

7) So to keep me from being too elated by the surpassing greatness of the revelations, a thorn was given me in the flesh, a messenger of Satan to harass me, to keep me from being too elated. 8) Three times I pleaded with the Lord about this, that it should leave me. 9) But he said to me, "My grace is sufficient for you, for my power is made perfect in weakness." Therefore I will boast all the more gladly of my weaknesses, so that the power of Christ may rest upon me. 10) For the sake of Christ, then, I am content with weaknesses, insults, hardships, persecutions, and calamities. For when I am weak, then I am strong.

Theme Verse: 2 Corinthians 12:9 "But he said to me, 'My grace is sufficient for you, for my power is made perfect in weakness.' Therefore I will boast all the more gladly of my weaknesses, so that the power of Christ may rest upon me."

Summary: 2 Corinthians is one of two letters written by the Apostle Paul to the community of believers living in the city of Corinth, located in Greece. Paul has had need to write them because of moral, ethical, relational and theological problems. Because they've not wanted to listen to what he had to say he has had to promote himself as a legitimate leader who has the authority to confront their problems. Yet in the very midst of promoting himself he also confessed personal and physical weaknesses in his life. He stated very clearly throughout 2 Corinthians that ultimately authority, abilities, strength and wisdom come from God and not from us.

Observation: There's probably no Biblical text more opposite of what all aspects of physical fitness are about than the verses in our reading for today. When was the last time you were in a weight room, cross-fit session, completing a marathon or attending zumba and you heard such statements as "power is made perfect in weakness" (vs. 9), "I will boast all the more gladly of my weaknesses" (vs. 9), "I am content with weaknesses" (vs. 10), and "when I am weak, then I am strong" (vs. 9) These are the last statements you'd ever hear in such settings. When I'm in the gym, the young men are flexing in front of the mirrors and making sure they're lifting more weight for a particular exercise than the last guy used. In the cross-fit session everyone's competing to be the one who lasts the full session without giving in to a rest. And so it goes, strength and endurance are essential aspects of fitness. Weakness like Paul talks about is the last thing to be exalted. But it's important to note this weakness seems to come from an affliction he calls "a thorn in the flesh." We don't know what it was, but he so disliked it that he prayed three times to get rid of it. But God had other plans for him. He knew it was best for Paul to have this affliction so that he would not be given to pride. After all, he was an important man in the life of the early church and it would have been easy for him to be prideful.

Application: It's very easy in the world of fitness to become prideful. We might think we aren't given to pride but if you're into weights, what do you do when you walk by a mirror? Probably flex and if no one's around even do some posing. Why do you wear tank tops and tight shirts? Probably to highlight the size and definition of your muscles. Why the tight leggings that hug the butt? To show the hours doing zumba are working. It's not wrong to be physically fit, have good-sized muscles, and be toned. We should be thankful that the hours spent involved in the exercises needed for these things are happening. What's wrong is being prideful about it. Pride generally means we think we're more important or better than someone else. Let's remember we are who we are and what we are like because of God's enabling. Struggling with pride? Maybe instead of praying like Paul did for his thorn to be removed we need to ask God to give us a thorn to keep us from exalting ourselves. Certainly this would be a novel idea. But remember the final words of Paul call us to a life content with who we are if it is "for the sake of Christ…" (vs. 10).

Day 31
Exercise – Good or Bad?

Biblical Text: 1 Timothy 4:1-16

1) Now the Spirit expressly says that in later times some will depart from the faith by devoting themselves to deceitful spirits and teachings of demons, 2) through the insincerity of liars whose consciences are seared, 3) who forbid marriage and require abstinence from foods that God created to be received with thanksgiving by those who believe and know the truth. 4) For everything created by God is good, and nothing is to be rejected if it is received with thanksgiving, 5) for it is made holy by the word of God and prayer.

6) If you put these things before the brothers, you will be a good servant of Christ Jesus, being trained in the words of the faith and of the good doctrine that you have followed. 7) Have nothing to do with irreverent, silly myths. Rather train yourself for godliness; 8) for while bodily training is of some value, godliness is of value in every way, as it holds promise for the present life and also for the life to come. 9) The saying is trustworthy and deserving of full acceptance. 10) For to this end we toil and strive, because we have our hope set on the living God, who is the Savior of all people, especially of those who believe.

11) Command and teach these things. 12) Let no one despise you for your youth, but set the believers an example in speech, in conduct, in love, in faith, in purity. 13) Until I come, devote yourself to the public reading of Scripture, to exhortation, to teaching. 14) Do not neglect the gift you have, which was given you by prophecy when the council of elders laid their hands on you. 15) Practice these things, devote yourself to them, so that all may see your progress. 16) Keep a close watch on yourself and on the teaching. Persist in this, for by so doing you will save yourself and your hearers.

<u>Theme Verse:</u> I Timothy 4:7 "...train yourself for godliness;"

<u>Summary:</u> The two books of Timothy contain the Apostle Paul's two letters to a young pastor named Timothy, who is pastoring a church in the city of Ephesus, which is located in present-day Turkey. Timothy is challenged by people in his church teaching different doctrine (ch.1 vs. 3). They are teaching that if you follow certain practices and teachings, you will become godly. Paul says the things they are teaching about spirits, demons, marriage, and food are not going to make you godly. Their thought was that if you avoided certain lifestyles (sex in marriage, and food), you would transform your life, but Paul steers them to a correct understanding. Our foundation for godliness and a better life come from

fixing our hope not on self, but on the living God (vs. 10).

Observation: Think about it. When you travel through airports and look at magazine stands or at these same stands in grocery stores or bookstores, what is being taught in sports and fitness magazines as the way to the good life? The good life comes from having a finely tuned body, massive arms, six-pack abs, or a slender waist and thighs. While it is good to be healthy and strong and have a low percentage of body fat, it does not necessarily change how you live each day or prepare you for life after death.

Application: Though Paul is correct when he says in verse 8 that "…bodily training is of some value," he is not saying it is of no value. In general, bodily exercise will affect your physical and emotional well-being. Bodily exercise can even affect your service. Have you ever traveled to Mexico to help build houses? I remember on my last building trip, having to carry hundreds of thirty-three pound cement blocks and pushing 800 wheelbarrows of cement. Had I not been relatively fit, I could not have effectively served the Lord on that mission trip. So continue or start to exercise, for it will affect your life, but do not believe the lies that teach the good life is only found in fitness.

Post-script

I hope that over the last thirty-one days, reading this devotional book, <u>Dual Fitness: Physical & Spiritual</u>, you have come to a foundational understanding of the importance of both physical and spiritual fitness. As God's creation it is so very important that we pursue both elements of fitness so that we can be all he intended us to be. Fitness, both physical and spiritual are things that have to be pursued all of our life. There will never be a time when you can sit back and say "I've achieved them, now I can coast." Neither physical nor spiritual fitness work this way. The day you coast is the day you begin to become unfit in both areas. Both need to be continually pursued. So, press on. Embrace physical fitness so you can enjoy the life God gives you to live; embrace spiritual fitness and enjoy the God who created you.

Blessings in your pursuit,
Daniel Grell

For any questions about physical fitness please see a local personal fitness trainer in your area.

For any questions about spiritual fitness contact Daniel at <u>havingagoodwalk@gmail.com</u>

For any speaking requests of the author or information about hosting a Dual Fitness retreat contact Daniel at <u>havingagoodwalk@gmail.com</u>

Scripture Index

Personal Reflections